Evidence

A Critical Reader

Evidence-Based General Practice
A Critical Reader

Leone Ridsdale, BA, MSc, PhD, FRCP(C)
Senior Lecturer and General Practitioner
Department of General Practice
UMDS of Guy's and St Thomas's Hospitals
London

W. B. Saunders Company Ltd
London Philadelphia Toronto Sydney Tokyo

W. B. Saunders   24–28 Oval Road
Company Ltd   London NW1 7DX

             The Curtis Center
             Independence Square West
             Philadelphia, PA 19106-3399, USA

             Harcourt Brace & Company
             55 Horner Avenue
             Toronto, Ontario, M8Z 4X6, Canada

             Harcourt Brace & Company, Australia
             30–52 Smidmore Street
             Marrickville
             NSW 2204, Australia

             Harcourt Brace & Company, Japan
             Ichibancho Central Building
             22–1 Ichibancho
             Chiyoda-ku, Tokyo 102, Japan

© 1995 W. B. Saunders Company Ltd

Second printing 1995
Fourth printing 1996

This book is printed on acid-free paper

All rights reserved. No part of this publication may be reproduced, stored in a retrieval system or transmitted, in any form or by any other means, electronic, mechanical, photocopying or otherwise, without the prior permission of W. B. Saunders Company Ltd, 24–28 Oval Road, London NW1 7DX.

A catalogue record for this book is available from the British Library

ISBN 0-7020-1611-X

Typeset by Phoenix Photosetting, Chatham, Kent
Printed and bound in Great Britain by
WBC Book Manufacturers Ltd, Bridgend

Contents

	Page
Preface	vii
Acknowledgements	ix
1. Introduction	1
2. Time for the Consultation	7
3. Making Sense of 'Minor' Illness	19
4. Patients' Ideas	27
5. Psychological Distress in General Practice	37
6. Communication During the Consultation	49
7. Screening for Carcinoma of the Cervix	59
8. Medical Ethics	77
9. The Economic Aspects of General Practice	86
10. Making Sense of Workload Studies	96
11. Diffusion of Innovation	106
12. Changing the Skill Mix in the Primary Care Team	119
13. Critical Appraisal	133
14. A Critical Appraisal of the Literature on Tiredness	148
15. How Do You Know? The Process of Scientific Reasoning	160
Appendices	170
Index	175

For Serife

Preface

I hope this book will provoke the reader to think critically about certain areas of general practice. In order to encourage a sense of debate, I have not tried to hide my own ideas and values. When I am enjoying reading a book myself, I write my own responses in the margin. I hope that this book encourages readers to write all over it.

It is not intended that the published evidence should be interpreted as 'facts'. I have tried to present it so that the reader considers all the topic areas as being continuously open to enquiry and debate. I want to foster an approach which challenges dogmatism, certainty and cosy consensus, without going over the top into a condemnation of some research evidence and practice or into paralyzing uncertainty. Having and recognizing one's own values is fine, but it is also important to expose oneself to counter-arguments and conflicting evidence (Evidence-Based Medicine Working Group, 1992).

If I had described and appraised the methods used in detail when discussing evidence on a particular topic, the arguments would have progressed rather slowly. So evidence has been presented 'on the hoof' and in a relatively uncritical way. However, later in the book there is a chapter on critical appraisal which draws on some of the evidence presented in previous chapters. The aim of this is to offer a simple framework for appraising papers. This approach to critical appraisal is applied subsequently to the literature on patients with 'tired all the time' syndrome. The final chapter draws back the camera lens to look at the construction of theories and their testing from the point of view of a historian or philosopher. I have left these more difficult topics to the end in the hope that the reader will be interested in reading about them after more practical questions have been debated.

How can a book like this hang together? This was a question that troubled me, since it was first raised by a publisher. Just as philosophers might define philosophy as whatever philosophers do, general practice could be defined as whatever GPs do. For me, general practice consists of a mixture of events, problems and challenges that are acted out in the space where patients' lives and needs overlap with my own. To understand this requires me to learn languages and gain insights offered by many specialist disciplines. Each of them offers different perspectives which do not necessarily cohere. General practice need not be reduced to one discipline or one framework for debate. The philosopher Rorty (1989) suggested that it is a misconception to try to fit everything together, whatever the subject. This philosophy of continuing to approach problems from different standpoints seems particularly appropriate when describing my thinking as a GP.

I could argue more simply that everyone strives to make meaning of what they do. This is my attempt. Some coherence may lie in there being one author. But my ideas have changed over the years of writing. The chapter on time was written first and had to be updated. The last chapter on the philosophy of science is still evolving as I continue to try to learn and understand more about my life and work.

Leone Ridsdale

References

Evidence-Based Medicine Working Group (1992). Evidence-based medicine: A new approach to teaching the practice of medicine. *Journal of the American Medical Association* 268: 2420–2425.

Rorty, R. (1989) *Contingency, Irony and Solidarity*. Cambridge: Cambridge University Press.

Acknowledgements

Writing a book can be solitary work, and can only be sustained with the support of family, friends and colleagues. The unsung heroes behind most writers are the librarians who patiently and diligently search for the references needed. Heather Lodge did this for me. Julia Shaw typed the manuscript and Suzanne Jeffrey checked the references. My publisher Georgina Bentlif provided support and all sorts of sensible advice.

Many friends and colleagues read a chapter or two, and a few generously gave the time to read it all the way through. I am immensely grateful for the critical feedback which was provided by Julie Beattie, Rob Caird, Peter Cantillon, Sean Coughlin, Ian Cromarty, John Ford, Fiona Gelder, John Horder, Sue Law, Myfanwy Morgan, Eileen Munro, Gerard Panting, David Sleator and Gillian Smith. I would also like to thank Ri Hornung who helped me apply for the prolonged study leave which gave me the time to finish writing.

The editors of the *British Medical Journal* and the *British Journal of General Practice* have given permission for their guidelines for referees to be published. I am grateful also to the examiners for the Royal College of General Practitioners for allowing questions from the *Critical Reading Paper* to be published here. Churchill Livingstone gave permission for me to quote from a chapter I wrote from *Screening and Surveillance in General Practice*, which was edited by Doctors Hart and Burke.

1
Introduction

This book is about some of the problems or topics arising in general practice. The topics are not necessarily the 'core topics', but some which I think are important. The choice of topics was difficult. Some were areas which have been researched quite extensively, for example, time and the consultation. Some have whole books written about them, such as medical ethics. Other topics are, in my opinion, important but little is written about them in the context of general practice, for example, the effect of economic incentives on doctors' behaviour. I have included them because I would like to see them on the agenda.

I now intend to describe some of the events and thoughts that occur to me in the course of a few working days. These will act as the substrate for discussion in the chapters which follow.

The names of the patients discussed have been changed to protect confidentiality.

Patients and my questions

My first patient had been fitted in at the beginning of the morning as an extra. As I did not know of this in advance, those who followed who had booked their appointment times were kept waiting. The problem of knowing how time should be allocated to suit the different and sometimes competing needs of patients, and how to optimize the use of the time that I have to offer, is my first challenge. The questions and some possible answers are discussed in Chapter 2.

My first patient was Mrs Smith and her 4-year-old son, Sean. She told me Sean had had a sore throat last week and that over the weekend he had developed an earache. She also had a cold. The Smiths have two small children and a third is on the way. Mr Smith has been warned that the firm he works for is to be closed down next year. During this consultation I pondered the many possible reasons for Mrs Smith attending then, and which ones I needed to focus on and manage on that day. These questions and some evidence is discussed in Chapter 3.

The next three patients were: a young mother whose 2-year-old had a cough; a hypertensive with a blood pressure of 200/120, whom the practice nurse suspected was not taking his pills; and a 30-year-old epileptic who lived in his parents' home. The fact that I was running behind made it difficult for me to enquire about the patients' views. I knew that if I did have the time, each of these patients would have a story to tell about their understanding of the problem. This information would have helped me to understand them and their behaviour. In-depth research involving interviews with patients like these might also help doctors to understand patients' ideas. Some of this qualitative research is described in Chapter 4.

The next patient came in and burst into tears. Through her tears she said that her husband was going to leave her and the children. Then Mr and Mrs Chard came in. He was losing weight quite rapidly due to his pancreatic cancer. Although the problem had been explained to him, he repeatedly asked for reassurance that he was getting better. His wife told me that he was angry and irritable at home, and asked if she could see a counsellor.

During our coffee break my trainee told me that he had reviewed the notes from the patients seen during the previous week. One of the things that struck him was that he had classified approximately one in ten of his patients as having psychological problems, whereas I had classified about one in five of the patients who consulted me in this way. He pointed out that the number of patients we saw in this period was relatively small, so this difference may have been a chance finding. We discussed why doctors may differ in their diagnosis and management of psychological problems. These issues are debated in Chapter 5.

Bearing in mind the patients I saw, their ideas and the constant shortage of time, it seems to me that one of the most important things about my work is the need to communicate as well as possible. There is a popular idea circulating among GPs that doctors in general practice are good at communicating with patients, and there are a number of models which demonstrate how this should be done. But how is it possible to tell whether GPs are good enough as communicators? Have they just developed a cosy consensus of opinion to make themselves feel good? I am not sure whether it is possible to test these ideas, and, if communication is thought to be important, how to test GPs. Models, measurement and learning about communication are discussed in Chapter 6.

After my coffee break I saw two patients with gynaecological problems. The first was a new patient called Mrs Dodds. She complained of bleeding after intercourse. She was 45 and lived in temporary council accommodation. She seemed to have moved house frequently. She told me that she had never received a letter inviting her for cervical screening. The second patient had had a smear and had been asked to return for a repeat in 6 months. 'What is mild dyskariosis?' she asked me. She told me that she had private medical insurance and asked if the problem was important enough for her to go privately sooner. I find the whole area of screening a really difficult one to make up my mind about, let alone advise patients on. In Chapter 7, some criteria for deciding on the effectiveness of screening are presented and applied to cervical cancer screening. Problems with the system and potential options for change are also considered.

The next person who came to see me was Mrs Black. She was not a patient of mine, but had asked me to see her so that we could talk about her 77-year-old mother-in-law, a patient of mine. Mrs Black explained that she and her husband were worried about my patient's ability to drive. She evidently did not turn on her headlights at night and sometimes could not find the pedals. Mrs Black said that her mother-in-law never used indicators. When she questioned her about this, her mother-in-law claimed that she did not need to use the indicators as *she* knew what she was going to do. Mrs Black and her husband had discussed their concerns with my patient but this had only led to some family friction and now they wanted me to do something about it. Next, a 44-year-old woman came to see me with a prescription for fertility drugs from a private doctor. She asked me to copy this onto an NHS prescription pad so that she could get the drugs at less expense. These problems led me to think about medical ethics and the law, issues which are discussed in Chapter 8.

Mr Metal was a 59-year-old lorry driver who came to see me with back pain which made it difficult for him to drive for long periods. I arranged for some physiotherapy, and when he developed a slight foot-drop I referred him to the local orthopaedic surgeon. The surgeon initially managed the problem conservatively, and then booked him for surgery, which was performed approximately a year later. Mr Metal's clinical condition was unchanged after the operation. At this consultation, we discussed the possibility of his taking early retirement. During the same period that I was looking after him, I was also seeing a patient with back pain who had private medical insurance. He had no neurological signs. He was referred to the same orthopaedic surgeon and was operated on a few weeks after his condition began. Thinking about these two cases led me to ruminate about the access patients have to medical care, and the efficiency and effectiveness of the service in dealing with their problems. This raises issues which are sometimes approached in different ways by specialists in ethics, economics and epidemiology. It is difficult to bring perspectives from these different disciplines to bear on a problem without first understanding the 'jargon' or specialist language. The aim of Chapter 9 is to introduce ideas and evidence about the uses of economics in planning and predicting medical activity.

After my surgery was over, I finished completing a questionnaire for the Department of Health on workload. Filling in the questionnaire for one week had been quite difficult. When I counted up the hours I worked, they totalled 75. And yet there is still an image in circulation of general practitioners not working particularly long hours, and having plenty of free time to spend on the proverbial golf course. Some of the reports of studies I have read in the past do not do much to change this popular image. The week in which I monitored my work seemed pretty typical for me, and I am not convinced that I was working much longer hours than my colleagues. This seeming disparity between the public image and private reality led me to look critically at the research published on workload. This is discussed in Chapter 10.

At lunch time I attended a meeting of the Medical Audit Advisory Group (MAAG). The Chairman had asked each of us to provide a summary of the previous year's work and the achievements in general terms of the practices we had visited. This led me to think about the locality in which I work. A few of my contemporaries among the local GPs had trained alongside me and many were in a young GP group with me. Since then, I have been a doctor to some and a patient to others. The role of Medical Audit Advisor has given me the opportunity to visit every practice in my area and discuss problems and progress with them. Some practices had recruited and trained nurses to a high level in the 1980s. Some had borrowed and invested enormous sums of money to create purpose-built surgeries. This had involved a considerable amount of debt and some risk when seen in context of falling prices on the housing market. Some practices had spent time and energy summarizing notes, and subsequently transferring information onto computers and learning how to use them during the consultation.

One of the fascinating aspects of those practice visits for me was that each partner in the practice had a different attitude to these changes. When I considered each of these individuals and what they had achieved together as a group, it made me want to know more about the process of change. I found that relatively little research had been done on this in British general practice. There was quite a lot of published evidence on the diffusion of innovation in America, and some of this described tradition and change in other areas such as agriculture. Chapter 11 explores the extent to which the theories and evidence about behaviour change described so far can help to explain what goes on in British general practice.

At the MAAG meeting, we discussed how the primary care team can meet the needs of patients who sometimes get ignored, for

Introduction

example, those with epilepsy. Everyone seems to be so overworked that it is difficult to imagine how we can improve care at the interface between hospitals and the community without changing the skill mix in the primary care team. Chapter 12 introduces the issues and evidence on this subject.

In the evening after work, I put my feet up and settled down to some reading. Earlier in the week I had been sent two papers, one by the *British Medical Journal* and one by the *British Journal of General Practice*. They were both on topics that interested me. The editors had asked my opinion about their suitability for publication, and each of them had included checklists of their criteria for eligibility. The process of appraising papers, and sometimes making suggestions as to how writers can clarify a description of what they have done, is challenging. It acts as a learning process. This experience has taught me what to look for and how to read between the lines of published work. Chapter 13 discusses some of the criteria I use in appraising papers and links these points with research that has been cited in the chapters preceding it.

The following morning I got up early. One of the journals which is distributed free to general practitioners had asked me to write a summary of the literature on tiredness. As it was a topic on which I had done a research project and reviewed the literature, I believed that I could meet the journal's deadline which was only a week away. In order to produce a summary of the clinical topic, I sifted through what had been written. The wheat which readers want is the evidence which might help them in clinical practice. The chaff, from the point of view of the journal editors and readers, is my evaluation of the process of the research project described, and the way that they can contextualize it within the research literature.

All practitioners must rely, to a certain extent, on other people to carry out this sifting process for them. We cannot sift through the literature on every topic and simultaneously practise in an area which brings together so many different specialities. However, some clinicians, particularly those who are actively learning or teaching or doing research, will periodically collect and go through the literature on certain topics. The process of sifting through the published evidence provides a learning process about why reviewers cite or omit to cite evidence from certain papers, and it enables the practitioner to understand to what extent particular questions have been answered or remain unanswered on a topic. Chapter 13 discusses this sifting skill, which is part of the process of collecting useful evidence, by going through some of the literature on tiredness.

Later on that day, I went to our local medical centre. A specialist was introduced, the lights were dimmed and he ran through his slides for 50 minutes. When he had finished, the lights went up, and the questions started. The audience of general practitioners were trying to relate their experience and questions to the evidence that had been presented to them. This made me ask myself: how do we as doctors justify our clinical reasoning? Each of us seems to have built up our beliefs in general practice based on a series of contingencies. We can see things from different standpoints and describe things in different ways. We often doubt the value of our plural approach, especially when confronted by notions like 'rational', 'logical' and 'objective'. Chapter 15 discusses how we claim to 'know' what is going on in science and in practice.

Some readers may be trainees or young GPs preparing for the Royal College of General Practitioners membership examinations, in particular the Critical Reading section. Many of the topics covered have been the subject of written or oral questions. In order to illustrate the type of questions asked, examples are given after the references at the end of the chapters. The guidelines for critical appraisal given to referees by the *British Medical Journal* and the *British Journal of General Practice* are also provided in the Appendices following the last chapter.

2

Time for the Consultation

> My first patient had been fitted in at the beginning of the morning as an extra. As I did not know of this in advance, the patients who had booked their appointment times were kept waiting. This was not an unusual surgery.

Introduction

I wondered whether audit and research about time and the consultation might help me to understand and manage my time better. Four particular aspects seemed likely to be relevant. The first is: what do patients want? Do they see the time spent waiting and the time the GP spends with them as important issues? Which patients are likely to be dissatisfied, and what problems do they have? What would patients like to see improved? And in what ways can they be improved?

The second aspect is: what are the professional and personal implications of the way in which doctors structure their time? Many general practitioners regard the consultation as central to their professional work and job satisfaction. But to what extent is the quality of communication dependent on time availability? If communication is time dependent, how do GPs divide time between patients? Some patients are more demanding than others, but presumably doctors try to divide up their time in proportion to patients' needs. To what extent do doctors distribute their time fairly?

I once worked in a practice where it was often necessary to see patients at 5 minute intervals. Our list size was large and so was our income. Remembering the stress and the lack of job satisfaction, I wonder if there is a general relationship between the rate at which doctors see patients and their stress level and feeling of job satisfaction.

The third aspect is the question of cost. An old aphorism is that 'time is money', and as the government is the purchaser of health care, cost is important. Does the time spent on consultations affect the use of other costly items, like drugs? I feel intuitively that when I make available more of what Balint (1957) called 'the drug doctor', I prescribe fewer of the conventional pharmacological remedies. I wonder if there is evidence to prove that the cost of more time spent on the consultation might be compensated for by less prescribing. Finally, how much time do doctors spend on average with their patients in other countries, and what are their costs?

My fourth concern is with better organization. How should doctors schedule their appointments? Can patients accurately identify the amount of time they need? How can appointment systems allow for the different needs of patients and the different abilities of doctors? Can a balance be reached between the patient's need for time and the time available to the doctor?

Thinking about time spent on the consultation raises many questions. Later, I looked through the published evidence to find out to what extent my questions could be answered. I know that researchers are just like GPs and can be prejudiced, so I looked carefully at the hypotheses and methods described by each investigator, before deciding on the importance to attach to their results. I also tried to identify the questions that remain unanswered which may be important for practice and research in future.

Patients' views and their level of satisfaction

It is difficult to generalize about patients' views, as patients vary just as much as their doctors do. Satisfaction with services will depend to a certain extent on expectations. Not only do patients differ, but expectations also change from one generation to the next. Over the years, expectations tend to increase. As a result, although the service may remain at approximately the same standard or even improve, satisfaction levels may fall.

Consumer groups and social scientists have tried to measure patients' views about their doctors and consultations. Cartwright and Anderson (1981) interviewed a sample of patients and their doctors in two surveys 14 years apart. They found that younger people and middle class patients were generally less satisfied than older people and working class patients. When patients were asked about the consultation process, the aspects most frequently criticized included the doctor:
1. not explaining things fully;
2. keeping people waiting in the waiting room;
3. taking too much time and not hurrying patients.

Time for the consultation

Have things changed since the second survey which was carried out in 1977? A more recent survey by the Consumer Council (Anon, 1989) found that patients stated that the most important improvement GPs could make would be to spend more time explaining about illness and more time listening to patients. A shorter wait at the surgery was also an important priority.

Patients clearly identify the length of time they spend waiting to see the doctor and the short time general practitioners make available for listening and explaining as less satisfactory parts of the service. But is there evidence that offering different appointment times can satisfy patients? Hull and Hull (1984) obtained information about the length of appointments offered by 25 doctors and measured the satisfaction levels reported by their patients. They found that dissatisfaction increased with shorter booked appointment times and vice versa. Younger patients and patients with psychological problems had higher dissatisfaction levels. More than 50% of women aged between 15 and 44 years reported difficulty in telling their doctor about their problem.

It appears from this descriptive study that when doctors offer shorter appointments their patients are less satisfied and vice versa. However, one cannot be sure that satisfaction levels are a direct consequence of the booking interval. Doctors who are more skilled as communicators may offer longer consultations, a characteristic which may confound the analysis. In order to test the hypothesis that the booking interval is directly related to patient satisfaction, it would be necessary to ask the same doctors to vary the booking interval and then measure patient satisfaction. Ridsdale and colleagues (1989) allocated 5, 10 or 15 minute consultations to patients in their practice. Significantly more patients reported they had too little or far too little time with the doctor in surgeries booked at shorter intervals.

To what extent does the amount of explanation doctors give depend on the time available in the consultation? Roland et al. (1986) and Ridsdale et al. (1989) varied appointment intervals in two practices and recorded GPs' statements explaining the patient's problem and suggested management, from approximately 1,500 consultations. In consultations booked at longer intervals, significantly more statements were made by the doctor explaining the problem and its management.

Counting statements of a particular kind is a simple measure of quality which can be used by trainees and GPs to observe and measure what they actually do. When GPs compare what they do, they sometimes find that what they actually do and omit to do is not what they would have expected. This simple audit technique could be used more widely.

Doctors' concerns
Communication

The consultation is regarded by most GPs as the kernel of their medical work. To what extent does time limit the level of communication possible? Verby and colleagues (1980) rated trainees' level of communication with their patients during the training year. They found that trainees increased the speed of their consultations during the course of their training. However, unless special teaching was provided using audiovisual feedback, their scores as communicators simultaneously declined. The same researchers (1979) also rated the consultations of two groups of experienced principals. One group reviewed their recorded interviews with a view to improving their performance. The scores which subsequently measured their communication improved significantly, but this was accompanied by a 40 per cent increase on time spent on the consultation.

This suggests that time, together with knowledge and skills, permits better communication to occur. In order to isolate the effect of time alone, Roland et al. (1986) and Ridsdale et al. (1989) measured the effect of increasing available appointment time on the interaction between doctors and patients. They found GPs asked more questions and facilitated the patient speaking more frequently in longer consultations. Ridsdale and colleagues (1992) subsequently demonstrated that individual doctors responded differently when more time was available. All the doctors asked more questions when more time was available. But doctors who did more facilitating than their colleagues in short consultations were more likely to increase their use of facilitation when more time was available. This supports the hypothesis that more time permits doctors to apply more frequently the communication behaviours they have already learned to practise. In Ridsdale's practice, patients also asked significantly more questions and expressed their own views more frequently when consultations were booked at longer intervals.

If time is important in determining consultation content, an important question is: how do doctors divide their time between different types of patients? Two descriptive studies by Buchan and Richardson (1973) and Bain (1976) measured the time and content of the consultation. Both studies found that slightly more time was given to middle class than to working class patients. Consultation analysis showed that middle class patients tended to present their symptoms more fully and ask more questions, and in turn they were given more advice by their GP.

More recent work by Boulton and others (1986) suggests a different picture. For this study, the researchers developed a sophisticated system of measuring what was said in the consultation, and then asked patients about the consultation afterwards. The results suggest that middle class patients were more active than working class patients in presenting their ideas to the doctor and seeking further explanation of their views. However, this did not necessarily mean that middle class patients got more benefit from the consultation. The investigators found that similar proportions of working class and middle class patients received explanations from the doctor, and similar proportions misunderstood and rejected the doctor's views and advice.

Diagnosis and management

Stott and Davis (1979) emphasized that doctors should ideally be able to address and cope with more than just the presenting problem. The additional agenda might include dealing with long-term health problems, health promotion and prevention, and psychosocial issues. Howie and colleagues (1991) asked doctors to time their surgeries and to note whether these areas had been identified and dealt with in consultations. Eighty-five GPs participated. The greatest differences were found in the number of psychosocial problems which were identified and dealt with. The number progressively increased with increased consultation length. As consultation length increased, the percentage of long-term problems doctors dealt with also increased significantly.

The investigators were able to identify differences between doctors in terms of their usual speed of consulting. But regardless whether they were usually fast or slow, doctors still recorded dealing with more psychosocial problems and more long-term health problems during longer consultations. It is not of course possible to say if this was partially due to the 'pull' effect of patient demand during these consultations. But doctors who generally consulted more slowly, consistently recorded the identification and management of more long-term and psychosocial problems.

Health promotion

Wilson and colleagues (1992) asked a group of GPs who were motivated to change to increase their consultation length. Sixteen GPs increased their average consulting time under experimental conditions from a median of 6 up to 7 minutes and recorded their health promotion activities. A proportion of the consultations were recorded, and patients were asked to complete a questionnaire about the topics raised. When more time was available during the consultation, both doctors and patients reported more discussion of smoking and measurement of blood pressure. When data from audiotapes were compared to doctors' records, it was found that doctors recorded only about half the health education they actually gave. This difference is perhaps not surprising to any busy doctor. But it also suggests that recorded observations of doctors' activities are likely to be more accurate than studies based on doctors' records alone.

Doctor stress and satisfaction levels

How are general practitioners affected emotionally by the pace at which they work, and does the pace at which they work affect their professional satisfaction? A survey by Calnan (1988) found that older, predominantly male doctors were more likely to have larger lists and see their patients in shorter consultations. Younger, more often female, doctors reported higher levels of work satisfaction. These GPs tended to have smaller lists and see their patients in longer consultations. Cooper and colleagues (1989) sent questionnaires to a different sample of doctors, enquiring about their job stress and satisfaction levels. The investigators found that older, male GPs reported more job stress and had higher anxiety levels than their colleagues. Women GPs had higher levels of job satisfaction. This evidence suggests that consultation behaviour may vary according to GPs' age, sex and financial needs, and this in turn may affect their job satisfaction.

When Wilson *et al.* (1991) asked general practitioners in one area to increase their available consultation time, 16 were motivated to do this and to measure their stress levels. Actual consultation time increased by a median of 1 minute, and waiting time for patients decreased from a median of 15 to 5 minutes. Under these circumstances, the GPs reported significantly less stress at the end of their surgeries.

Howie and colleagues (1992) also measured stress levels in their large study and linked them to the doctor's expressed attitude to medical care and his or her usual consulting speed. Doctors who had a more patient-orientated attitude were more likely to report more stress, spend more time on the consultation and deal with more psychosocial issues. When doctors whose preferred style was to consult slowly had to see more patients in a short period, they became even more stressed.

The area of doctors' attitudes, behaviour, stress and satisfaction levels is complex, but observations from studies using different designs do produce some common threads. It appears that doctors' age, sex, financial and professional expectations influence their behaviour during the consultation, and that this in turn generates different levels of stress and satisfaction or dissatisfaction with the work. Perhaps the most intractable difficulty for GPs is sharing not only their costs, but also the income they generate as a group.

Partners may impose a uniform consultation interval, so that in theory the workload will be evenly shared. Howie and his colleagues' results elegantly demonstrated the effect of forcing round pegs into square holes. When short of time, doctors who are usually patient-centred become stressed, and when under pressure give up trying to cover the potential areas which Stott and Davis (1979) described for every consultation.

Practice costs

Considering GP services in the aggregate leads to more precise questions about patient and doctor numbers. Can the time interval at which doctors see patients be related to the number of patients they can each manage? Morrell and Roland (1987) devised this formula:

Total consulting time = list size × consultation rate × duration of consultation

They found that consultation rate varied, but the average frequency was 3.5 consultations per patient per year. They calculated that if GPs retained their current total hours of work whilst wanting to spend on average 10 minutes on the consultation, they would need to reduce their list sizes to between 1,500 and 1,750 patients.

It is important to work these figures out in order to estimate the consequences of a change in national or local strategy. Some GPs may want to spend more time with their patients, and they may accept the implication that they will need to have fewer patients and possibly earn less, whilst other GPs may give priority to maximizing their income. Is there evidence that this occurs already?

Calnan (1988) asked doctors about their attitudes to their work and collected information about their list sizes and the time they spent on average on the consultation. He found that some doctors were more likely to say that their behaviour was influenced by financial incentives. This group spent on average less time on the consultation and had, on average, a larger list size. On the other hand, Calnan found that some doctors gave less priority to financial incentives. These doctors took a more psychosocial view of patients and were more likely to offer health education and screening. They spent more time on the consultation and had, on average, a smaller list size. It is difficult to draw inferences about the effect of change from a cross-sectional study like this one. In future, the relationship between doctors' attitudes and behaviour needs to be studied intermittently using qualitative as well as quantitative techniques.

Prescribing costs

A common belief is that if GPs spend more time on the consultation they will be able to prescribe less. Perhaps the things doctors provide, such as time or prescriptions, are to some extent substitutable. Is there any evidence to suggest this is so? Hughes (1983) compared two group practices working in a single health centre. Practice A normally booked consultations at 10 minute intervals, and practice B normally arranged consultations at 5 minute intervals. Hughes found a markedly lower proportion of consultations ending with a prescription in practice A. This supports the idea that practices offering longer consultations will prescribe less.

However, there were likely to be other important differences between the doctors in the two practices. The doctors' attitudes were likely to be different, and this may have affected both the time they made available and their prescribing patterns. The way to test this possibility would be for a group of doctors to agree to consult at varying intervals and then to measure their prescribing rate. Morrell and colleagues (1986) non-systematically allocated 5, 7.5 and 10 minute appointments to patients with doctors in one practice. They found that there was no evidence that patients who attended sessions booked at shorter intervals received more prescriptions. It is difficult to draw conclusions from this result. It is possible that some doctors who choose to give more time to each patient also choose to prescribe less. This hypothesis is supported by Howie et al.'s (1992) study. They measured doctors' attitudes to medical care and used the responses to classify 80 doctors as more or less 'patient-centred'. Doctors with a more positive attitude towards dimensions like psychological and preventive medicine spent more time on average on consultations and prescribed less.

National costs

As 'time is money', any increase in the time spent with patients will concern both the providers of health care (doctors) and the purchaser (the government), as well as patients. In order to achieve an equitable distribution of medical care, GPs generally accept the Government's monopoly position as purchaser of their services. But if doctors spent more time with their patients in the consultation, other compensatory changes would need to occur. For example, if total working hours were not to increase, GPs could spend less time on home visiting. Alternatively, GPs could increase their hours of work, resulting in an effective reduction in their income for the hours worked. But if doctors' hours and income were to remain in the same proportion, an increase in time spent on the consultation would cost the Government more to pay for the increase in time, and more doctors might need to work as GPs.

What happens elsewhere? In the United States and France, patients spend 14 minutes on average with their GP in the consultation, and doctors go on home visits much less frequently than in Britain (Sandier, 1990). Remuneration in these countries is not by an annual sum per patient (capitation) but by a fee for each appointment. Some patients shop around for medical advice, therefore increasing demand through duplication of services. Some doctors may ask patients to come back unnecessarily, to boost their own income. Reimbursement on a fee for service basis involves more administration. It is not surprising to find that overall the cost of health care per patient is much higher in these countries. But it is difficult to draw conclusions from comparing different countries, as countries differ in many other ways. Nevertheless, when changes are considered in the system of delivering medical care, doctors need to know about the models used elsewhere. This is important when deciding what to do and, just as importantly, what to avoid doing.

Providers and purchasers of health care have to make decisions about competing priorities. If patient satisfaction and service cost are directly associated, the aims of higher satisfaction and cost containment will necessarily be in conflict. At a small-scale 'micro' level, doctors who maximize patient satisfaction may do so at the expense of higher practice costs and lower income, and vice versa. At a national or 'macro' level, extreme patient dissatisfaction may cause governments to lose popularity with voters. But tax reductions are generally welcomed by voters, so voters are also endorsing cost containment. In a nationally controlled system, government decision-making must therefore balance the aim of cost containment against the limiting constraint of consumer dissatisfaction.

Organizing the booking system

Having considered the patients' view, doctors' personal and professional concerns, and cost, there are also organizational issues to work out. Do patients have a part to play in choosing their own appointment length? Can they accurately identify the amount of time they need? If they could do this, it might increase autonomy and consumer choice. What information is there about patients' ability to estimate their own needs? Lowenthal and Bingham (1987) offered their patients a choice of 5, 10 or 15 minute consultations. The doctors were not told of the interval the patient had chosen, but they measured the actual consultation length with a stopwatch. The investigators found that the mean consultation lengths were 6.5, 9.2 and 14.5 minutes, suggesting that patients are generally good at estimating the time they require. However, patients with a diagnosis of psychiatric disorder were less accurate in their choice of time. These patients often required more time than was scheduled for them, so the problem of how to reduce the waiting time for those booked after them remains.

Harrison (1987) introduced a system whereby patients estimated how much time they would need, and then he measured the waiting time for both patient and doctor. He found that when he compared this system to the old system of booking patients at 10 minute intervals, he was able to reduce patients' average waiting time from 6.3 minutes to 3.1 minutes, whilst the average waiting time for the doctor increased from 0.43 minutes to 0.67 minutes.

The challenge in devising an appointment system is to achieve a balance between the time the doctor waits for patients to arrive and the time the patient spends waiting to be seen. An appointment system can never achieve an exact balance, because of unforeseen problems, such as patients with psychological problems and medical emergencies. But it is possible for every doctor to determine an optimal booking interval, given his or her own average consulting speed. In order to do this, GPs need to be clear about the value which they attach to their own time, compared with their patients' time. Some doctors may find this difficult. And yet a desire to avoid gaps between patients has in the past caused patients to wait for an unnecessarily long time, the delays increasing as surgeries proceeded. This process may unwittingly cause doctors to rush consultations and give less than full attention to the patient.

Marshall (1986) and Hill-Smith (1989) have devised computer systems with which doctors could measure their average consultation length, doctor waiting time and patient waiting time, and calculate their optimal booking interval. Using a computer program, Hill-Smith was able to show that the doctor's waiting time was virtually nil until the appointment interval was increased to his average consulting speed, and then his waiting time increased linearly. For the patient, decreasing the appointment time to below the doctor's average consulting speed increased waiting time exponentially. Hill-Smith suggested that more frequent, shorter surgeries would result in less waiting time for patients, with no increase in the doctor's waiting time per consultation.

When I measured my own average consultation length, it was 8–9 minutes. One option for me was to book patients at 10 minute intervals in the morning from 9–10 a.m. and then again from 10.30–11.30 a.m. This allowed me 1–2 minutes between patients for writing notes and clearing my mind, which Neighbour (1987) described as housekeeping. If patients over-run their booking time, there is time to catch up after each hour's batch of appointments. If patients come without an appointment they can sometimes be fitted into the 10–10.30 a.m. interval, without increasing delays for those patients who have booked an appointment. If no additional patients need to be fitted in, this time can be used for administrative work. The research described so far was done before desktop computers. I know that using a computer affects the way I communicate, use of time during the consultation, and it affects the patient's view of me (Ridsdale and Hudd, 1994). Investigations of this new area will in turn affect how GPs teach and practise in the future.

References

Anon (1989) Doctor, doctor: What do you want from your GP? *Which* 481–483.
Bain, D. J. G. (1976) Doctor–patient communication in general practice consultations. *Medical Education* 10: 125–131.
Balint, M. (1957) *The Doctor, his Patient and the Illness*. London: Pitman.
Boulton, M., Tuckett. D., Olson, C. & Williams, A. (1986) Social class and the general practice consultation. *Sociology of Health and Illness* 8: 325–350.
Buchan, I. C. & Richardson, I. M. (1973) Time study of consultations in general practice. *Scottish Health Service Studies*, no. 27. Edinburgh: Scottish Home and Health Department.
Calnan, M. (1988) Images of general practice: The perceptions of the doctor. *Social Science and Medicine* 27: 579–586.
Cartwright, A. & Anderson, R. (1981) *General Practice Revisited*. Tavistock Publications Limited, London.
Cooper, C. L., Rout, U. & Faragher, B. (1989) Mental health, job satisfaction and job stress among general practitioners. *British Medical Journal* 298: 366–370.
Harrison, A. T. (1987) Appointment systems: Feasibility study of a new approach. *British Medical Journal* 294: 1465–1466.
Hill-Smith, I. (1989) Mathematical relationships between waiting times and appointment interval for doctor and patients. *Journal of the Royal College of General Practitioners* 39: 492–494.
Howie, J. G. R., Porter, A. M. D., Heaney, D. L. & Hopton, J. L. (1991) Long to short consultation ratio: A proxy measure of quality of care for general practice. *British Journal of General Practice* 41: 48–54.
Howie, J. G. R., Hopton, J. L., Heaney, D. L. & Porter, A. M. D. (1992) Attitudes to medical care, the organization of work, and stress among general practitioners. *British Journal of General Practice* 42: 181–185.
Hughes, D. (1983) Consultation length and outcome in two group general practices. *Journal of the Royal College of General Practitioners* 33: 143–147.
Hull, F. M. & Hull, F. S. (1984) Time and the general practitioner: The patient's view. *Journal of the Royal College of General Practitioners* 34: 71–75.

Lowenthal, L, & Bingham, E. (1987) Length of consultation: How well do patients choose? *Journal of the Royal College of General Practitioners* 37: 498–499.

Marshall, E. I. (1986) Waiting for the doctor. *British Medical Journal* 292: 993–995.

Morrell, D. C. & Roland, M. O. (1987) How can good general practitioner care be achieved? *British Medical Journal* 294: 161–162.

Morrell, D. C., Evans, M. E., Morris, R. W. & Roland, M. O. (1986) The 'five-minute' consultation: Effect of time constraint on clinical content and patient satisfaction. *British Medical Journal* 292: 870–873.

Neighbour, R. (1987) *The Inner Consultation*. Lancaster: MTP Press Limited.

Ridsdale, L. & Hudd, S. (1994) Computers in the consultation: The patient's view. *British Journal of General Practice* 44: 367–369.

Ridsdale, L., Carruthers, M., Morris, R. & Ridsdale, J. (1989) Study of the effect of time availability on the consultation. *Journal of the Royal College of General Practitioners* 39: 488–491.

Ridsdale, L., Morgan, M. & Morris, R. (1992) Doctors' interviewing technique and its response to different booking time. *Family Practice* 9: 57–60.

Roland, M. O., Bartholomew, J., Courtenay, M. J. F., Morris, R. W. & Morrell, D. C. (1986) The 'five-minute' consultation: Effect of time constraint on verbal communication. *British Medical Journal* 292: 874–876.

Sandier, S. (1990) Health services utilization and physician income trends. In: *Organisation for Economic Co-operation and Development Health Care Systems in Transition: The Search for Efficiency*. Paris: OECD.

Stott, N. C. H. & Davis, R. H. (1979) The exceptional potential in each primary care consultation. *Journal of the Royal College of General Practitioners* 29: 201–5.

Verby, J. E., Holden, P. & Davis, R. H. (1979) Peer review of consultations in primary care: The use of audio-visual recordings. *British Medical Journal* 1: 1686–1688.

Verby, J. E., Davis, R. H. & Holden, P. (1980) A study of the interviewing skills of trainee assistants in general practice. *Patient Counselling and Health Education* 68–71.

Wilson, A., McDonald, P., Hayes, L. & Cooney, J. (1991) Longer booking intervals in general practice: Effects on doctors' stress and arousal. *British Journal of General Practice* 41: 184–187.

Wilson, A., McDonald, P., Hayes, L. & Cooney, J. (1992) Health promotion in the general practice consultation: A minute makes a difference. *British Medical Journal* 304: 227–230.

Royal College of General Practitioners (RCGP) Examination Question

Outline and evaluate recent evidence supporting longer consultations in general practice. Critical Reading Paper, 6 May 1992.

3

Making Sense of 'Minor' Illness

> Mrs Smith brings her 4-year-old son, Sean, to the surgery. She says he had a sore throat last week and over the weekend he has developed an earache. She also has a cold. The Smiths have two small children and a third is on the way. Mr Smith has been warned that the firm he works for is to be closed down next year.

Introduction

Many of the problems patients bring to general practitioners are minor and self-limiting. Respiratory infections in children form a large part of this work. GPs may regard some of this work as trivial (Cartwright and Anderson, 1981). This raises a number of issues: why do patients seek help for minor problems? How do doctors manage these problems? Is there a 'scientific approach' to management?

Why do patients consult?

Uncommon symptoms

Morrell and Wale (1976) and Banks *et al.* (1975) made a detailed study of approximately 200 women patients who were between 20 and 44 years of age. The patients were asked to complete a health diary for a period of 4 weeks during the study year, and information was collected on who initiated consultations together with details of symptoms and diagnoses made during the same year.

Extrapolating from the diary experience, the investigators estimated that the women experienced about 80 episodes of symptoms per year, but on average initiated a consultation once for every 37 symptom episodes recorded. The researchers were able to relate the type of symptoms experienced to those presented during the consultations.

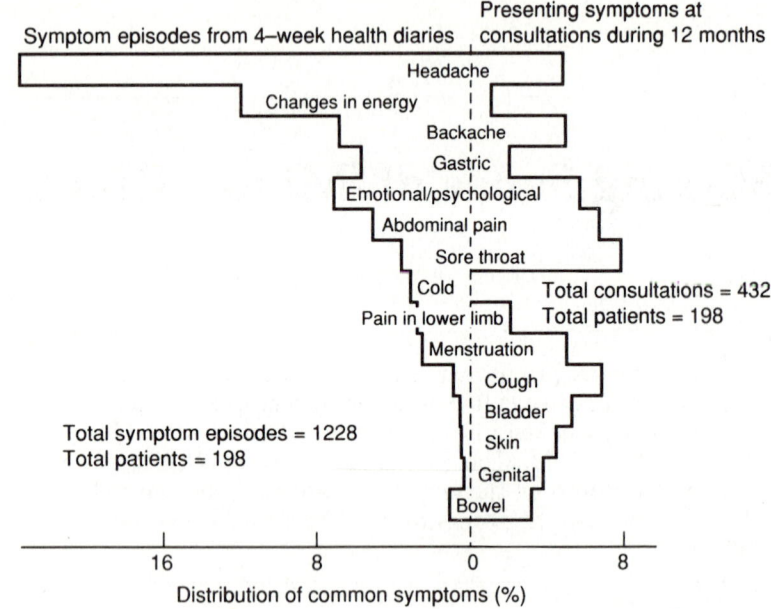

Fig. 3.1 Relationship between episodes of symptoms recorded in health diaries and symptoms presented at consultations. (From Banks *et al.*, 1975. By permission of Oxford University Press.)

According to the graphical representation, it appears that symptoms which are extremely commonly experienced are less likely to lead to a consultation than those which are less frequently reported. Headache and a change in energy levels were experienced frequently but they were presented less often to doctors. Sore throats and coughs were experienced less frequently but were more likely to lead to a consultation with the doctor. Thus, different symptoms seem to be evaluated differently by patients in terms of a decision to consult, and the frequency of occurrence of the symptoms is one factor which seems to affect the decision to seek help.

Severity

Part of the reason why a patient decides to consult a doctor may depend on the symptom being experienced less frequently. The decision may also depend on the perceived severity of the symptom. Ingham and Miller (1979) studied patients consulting and the severity of common symptoms reported at one health centre, and compared them with a control group on the practice list who had not seen their general practitioner. The investigators compared symptom severity between attenders who reported one or more of seven selected symptoms, and non-attenders who reported that they were troubled by the same symptoms. Symptoms like backache and tiredness were extremely common in both attending patients and in the comparison group, and had often lasted for a considerable period of time. But the investigators found that symptom severity was significantly greater in those who had consulted their doctor recently.

Anxiety

Unusual and severe symptoms are clearly related to the decision to consult, but some patients still consult more than others. Morrell and Wale (1976) and Banks et al. (1975) found that patients with higher scores on measures of anxiety were more likely both to record symptoms and to present them to their doctors.

The mental state of mothers is likely to be associated not only with their perception and management of their own symptoms, but also with their perception and management of symptoms experienced by other members of the family. This hypothesis was tested by Leach and his colleagues prospectively (1993). They asked mothers of young children to complete the General Health Questionnaire (GHQ) 28 which measures symptoms of depression and anxiety. They found that high anxiety scores in mothers were correlated with increased consultation frequency both for the mothers themselves and for their children.

Stress and life events

Anxiety levels may affect both people's perception of their symptoms and their tendency to consult with those symptoms. This anxiety may or may not be linked to external causative factors, but stress may be understood to arise as a consequence of external stressors. A relationship between social life events and psychological disease was proposed by Brown and Harris (1978). Stress in family groups may predispose family members to physical problems such as infections, and this may increase the frequency with which they consult. Meyer and Haggerty (1962) selected 16 families of similar socio-economic status, all of whom had two or more children, and studied them prospectively over the course of a year. These families were chosen because they were known to be high or low frequency consulters. The investigators conducted a series of interviews with the families and asked them to keep a diary of illness, therapy and life events. In addition, the researchers cultured samples taken from the throats of all family members every 3 weeks and tested for group A beta-haemolytic streptococcus.

Every 4 months they measured antistreptolysin-O titres in the blood.

Meyer and Haggerty (1962) found that 21 per cent of the throat cultures tested positive for beta-haemolytic streptococci, but less than half of the individuals who had positive cultures became ill. By looking at family diaries, the investigators found that streptococcal acquisition and subsequent illness was four times as likely to occur after than before stressful events. They also found that chronic stress was an important factor leading to illness when an individual was exposed to infection. After the acquisition of streptococci, a rise in antistreptolysin-O titres was seen in 21 per cent of patients in low stress families, compared to 49 per cent of patients in moderate to high stress families. The number of families was small, but the idea and design for the study was remarkable in attempting to test the hypothesis that those who perceived themselves as experiencing acute and chronic stress were more susceptible to developing physical illness when exposed to infection.

Cohen and co-workers (1991) took 395 healthy subjects and exposed them to virus infections under experimental conditions, while simultaneously asking them to complete self-assessment questionnaires measuring psychological stress levels. The investigators found that the rates of both respiratory infection and clinical colds increased in a dose–response manner in line with increases in the degree of reported psychological stress. This experiment was performed under controlled circumstances and supports the idea that although exposure to infectious agents is a prerequisite for illness, it is stress that in some way suppresses resistance, leaving individuals susceptible to physical illness.

Anxious individuals perceive life events and difficulties as being more stressful than other people do. This makes stress difficult to analyze, as the influence of life events, psychological states and subjective reports of symptoms are closely linked. But can objectively measurable life events and difficulties actually make people more vulnerable to illness and more likely to visit the doctor? Beale and Nethercote (1985) looked at the relationship between the threat of redundancy and patients' frequency of attending in one practice. They designed a case-control retrospective study in which patients who were made redundant by a factory closure were compared to patients who remained fully employed during the study period. The investigators found a significant increase in the frequency with which family members in the study group attended the surgery, and in the frequency with which they were referred on to hospital outpatient departments for physical as well as psychological conditions.

These changes in families' behaviour were found to have started 2 years before the actual job loss, at a time when a family member first learned that his or her job was in jeopardy. It is difficult to be sure that an increase in service use, that is, visits to the GP or a specialist, is necessarily the same thing as morbidity. Beale and Nethercote's study (1985) demonstrated how a life event, in this case the same event happening for a group of people within one community, influenced the number of consultations with GPs and specialists, and it showed that socio-economic factors are associated with medical work.

JRCGP

What should doctors do?

In the vignette that introduced this chapter a child was presented with a sore throat and earache, in the context of family stress and socio-economic disadvantage. In this situation, the doctor may get a strong sense from the patient or his mother of the feeling that something 'must be done'. In this context, the variation in doctors' responses have often been interpreted from a biomedical standpoint as being non-scientific. But a doctor's range of influence in this bio-social context is relatively small. New jobs and better housing cannot be prescribed, but an antibiotic can. The something that 'must be done' may therefore focus on the decision as to whether or not to prescribe.

What evidence is there that this kind of medical intervention helps? Burke and co-workers (1991) undertook a prospective double blind trial to test the comparative effectiveness of amoxycillin versus a placebo on 232 children. They reported that 'treatment failure' occurred, by which they meant a second antibiotic prescription was required eight times more frequently in the group given the placebo than in the group treated with antibiotics. Children in the placebo group also showed a significantly higher incidence of fever on the day after entry and an increased consumption of analgesics, mean duration of crying and mean length of absence from school.

BMJ

What do doctors do?

A patient's decision to consult may depend on many factors:
1. their assessment of the frequency of the symptom;
2. their perception of its severity;
3. their anxiety;
4. the occurrence of life events with social and economic implications for the family and their ability to cope with acute and chronic stress in their lives.

Doctors' responses need to be examined in this context. Howie (1976) decided to measure, in an experimental way, the extent to

BMJ

which doctors' knowledge of social and psychological data about the family influenced in their management policy of physical problems. He wrote to 1,000 general practitioners, sending them photographs of sore throats presented by patients, whilst varying the psychosocial information which was provided. He found that when additional data suggested that the individual or family was experiencing life events and difficulties which placed them under stress, GPs were significantly more likely to say that they would prescribe an antibiotic for a sore throat. Doctors were also more likely to state that they would prescribe when it might lead to more problems for patients or for doctors if the symptoms did not resolve quickly. For example, doctors were more likely to prescribe when the patient was planning to go on holiday the following week, or when the patient lived a long way from the practice.

Howie's experiment (1976) showed that GPs reported that they did respond to psychosocial factors when they prescribed for a physical complaint. Do doctors behave this way in practice? Howie and Bigg (1980) identified mothers who either had or had not been prescribed psychotropic drugs, and related this to the frequency with which these mothers brought their children to the doctor with respiratory tract infections. Mothers who had been classed as high psychotropic users were more likely to bring their children with acute respiratory illness, and these children were more likely to receive antibiotic drugs over a 10-year period. But when these data were plotted over time, it was found that these mothers were less likely to be receiving psychotropic drugs at times when their children were in receipt of antibiotic medication. Families receiving more treatment were also more likely to be living in council houses. Bain and Sales (1981) explored the bio-social connection in another way. They examined case notes in order to explore the relationship between mothers' consulting behaviour and the rate of referral of their children to an ear, nose and throat (ENT) department over a 5-year period. They found that when mothers consulted more themselves and received psychotropic drugs, their children were more likely to be referred to the ENT department. However, these children were less likely to be selected for surgery than children referred whose mothers were not receiving drugs. The investigators found that the practices they studied with the largest numbers of patients in the lower social classes had higher percentages of mothers receiving psychotropic drugs and higher referrals of children to ENT surgeons.

The results of these studies support the idea that patients' and doctors' behaviour is not determined solely by their perception of physical problems. Behaviour also varies according to social, psychological and economic influences. On the basis of these measurements, it is difficult to know precisely what is going on, or indeed what should be going on. One inference is that children of mothers who are in some way 'inadequate' or 'not coping' are over-medicalized. However, it is not possible to know from retrospective studies whether the children of mothers who received psychotropic medication were as ill as or more ill than other children. The data suggest that these families were more economically disadvantaged. In this case, there may have been other risk factors for respiratory infections, such as sharing rooms and living with parents who were smokers. In lower socio-economic groups, mothers are also more likely to be experiencing adverse life events and difficulties. These risk factors could lead to an increase in the incidence and severity of respiratory infections in the family, so it might be appropriate for the GP to treat both the mother *and* the child.

References

Bain, D. J. G. & Sales, C. M. (1981) Referring children to an ENT department and prescribing psychotropic drugs to their mothers. *British Medical Journal 283:* 585–587.

Banks, M. H., Beresford, S. A., Morrell, D. C., Waller, J. J. & Watkins, C. J. (1975) Factors influencing demand for primary medical care in women aged 20–44 years: A preliminary report. *International Journal of Epidemiology 4:* 189–195.

Beale, N. & Nethercote, S. (1985) Job-loss and family morbidity: A study of a factory closure. *Journal of the Royal College of General Practitioners 35:* 510–514.

Brown, G. W. & Harris, T. O. (1978) *Social Origins of Depression.* London: Tavistock Publications.

Burke, P., Bain, J., Robinson, D. & Dunleavey, J. (1991) Acute red ear in children: Controlled trial of non-antibiotic treatment in general practice. *British Medical Journal 303:* 558–562.

Cartwright, A. & Anderson, R. (1981) *General Practice Revisited.* London: Tavistock Publications Limited.

Cohen, S., Tyrell, D. & Smith, A. P. (1991) Psychological stress and susceptibility to the common cold. *New England Journal of Medicine 325:* 606–612.

Howie, J. G. R. (1976) Clinical judgment and antibiotic use in general practice. *British Medical Journal 2:* 1061–1064.

Howie, J. G. R. & Bigg, A. R. (1980) Family trends in psychotropic and antibiotic prescribing in general practice. *British Medical Journal 280:* 836–838.

Ingham, J. G. & Miller, P. McC. (1979) Symptom prevalence and severity in a general practice population. *Journal of Epidemiology and Community Health 33:* 191–198.

Leach, J., Ridsdale, L. & Smeeton, N. (1993) Is there a relationship between a mother's mental state and consulting the doctor by the family? *Family Practice 10:* 305–311.

Meyer, R. J. & Haggarty, R. J. (1962) Streptococal infections in families. *Paediatrics 29:* 539–549.

Morrell, D. C., Wale, C. J. (1976) Symptoms perceived and recorded by patients. *Journal of the Royal College of General Practitioners 26:* 398–403.

RCGP Examination Questions

Discuss the evidence concerning the role of antibiotics in treating otitis media in children. Critical Reading Paper, 6 May 1992.

Unemployment makes you ill'. Evaluate the evidence to support this statement. Critical Reading Paper, 29 October 1993.

4

Patients' Ideas

> A young mother brings her 2-year-old son with a cough.

> Our practice nurse asked me to see a patient because his blood pressure was 200/120. She suspected he had not been taking his pills.

> The next patient was a 30-year-old epileptic who lived with his mother.

Introduction

As doctors have spent many years training to think about and advise on medical conditions, there are differences between doctors' and patients' views. These differences in the meanings and explanations attached to illnesses may lead to misunderstandings if doctors inform and advise patients without asking patients what they themselves think about their own condition. Understanding patients' beliefs and behaviour is particularly important when trying to negotiate with patients about changes in their behaviour. This chapter will describe some of the literature on lay beliefs and behaviour, using the examples of cough, hypertension and epilepsy.

When investigating areas where little is known or conditions and behaviours are stigmatized, an in-depth, interviewing approach is a particularly useful way of learning more about the problem. Knowledge gained by this method can help doctors become aware of hidden ideas and concerns, so they can be raised and discussed during the consultation. This requires time and skill, as discussed in Chapters 2 and 6. The results of in-depth interviews are important sources of knowledge about concerns which are sometimes held as painful secrets by our patients.

An acute condition – cough

The most common reason for patients consulting their doctor is a respiratory complaint (RCGP, OPCS and DHSS, 1986). Children, boys in particular, are more likely to present with respiratory complaints. Respiratory complaints account for approximately one-quarter of consultations with doctors. The consultation rate for respiratory infections is highest in the youngest age groups. Doctors may regard some of these consultations as trivial and inappropriate.

A study of patients' beliefs provides a completely different perspective. Cornford and his colleagues (1993) interviewed a group of mothers who had consulted a general practitioner because their child had a cough. Initially, open-ended interviews were undertaken with a pilot group of mothers. From this, a schedule of open questions was derived, and 30 mothers were subsequently interviewed. Interviews were tape recorded, transcribed and analyzed so that the themes could be identified.

Twenty-two of the 30 mothers expressed concern that their child was going to die. Approximately half thought that their child might choke to death. These concerns were experienced at night in particular. One mother said:

'I wasn't sleeping, I was sleeping but I kept waking up, sort of every hour, every half hour, just thinking, just the thoughts, but it was just I couldn't rest, I was worried and it was affecting my sleep, yes, even though he wasn't awake. Yes, it was just a constant worry and, you know, you feel a bit foolish going to a doctor and saying, you know, I am not really saying to the doctor how you really feel, you know I sort of went in quite blasé, 'Oh, by the way, he has got a bit of a cough, is he all right?' where in fairness I am thinking, 'Is my child going to live?' Basically that is what I want to know. Is he going to survive this?' (Cornford et al., 1993).

Two-thirds of the mothers were concerned that the cough symptom was somewhere within the chest. Half of them believed that it might progress to a kind of permanent lung damage. One of them said:

'By watching his mama and nanna, you know being bad all the time with her chest and she can't catch her breath and with the bad weather and everything I don't want him to be like that when he gets older, I thought well it is best to treat it now and then he will be all right when he is older.' (Cornford et al., 1993).

The majority of mothers (25 out of 30) had tried proprietary medicines before taking their child to the doctor; the average number of medicines tried was 1.8 per child. Mothers often remarked, sometimes with disbelief, that whereas the cold appeared chesty to them, the doctor said the chest was clear after listening with a stethoscope.

Results from in-depth interviews such as these illustrate that the ideas and concerns patients bring to the consultation are sometimes far more serious than doctors might expect. A way of exploring this issue with a larger sample is by using structured questionnaires. Campion and Gabriel (1985) compared the cough characteristics of those who went to see the doctor with those who did not. They concluded that the severity of the child's illness, in particular the child needing more attention, experiencing difficulty in breathing, pain when coughing and sleeping during the day, determined whether consultation took place or not. This study was useful for focusing on differences between attenders and non-attenders and for providing information about the views of a larger group of mothers.

A chronic condition – hypertension

Hypertension is a risk factor for stroke, and stroke is the third largest cause of mortality in the UK (OPCS, 1993). Black people with hypertension are likely to have a poorer prognosis than white people. But apart from such general associations hypertension is an enigmatic condition. It may be asymptomatic. The cause is in most cases unknown, and even the words used to describe it mean different things to different people.

Blumhagen (1980) interviewed 103 patients attending a hospital-based hypertension clinic in North America. These patients had their blood pressure managed by nurse practitioners, and Blumhagen compared the patients' and the providers' views. When he interviewed the patients, he found that half of them attributed the cause of their condition to psychosocial problems. They said they had experienced a catastrophe in their lives which had precipitated the condition, or that they had long-standing work or family difficulties. One patient said:

'My interpretation is Hyper-Tension moves into high blood pressure and causes high blood pressure.' (Blumhagen, 1980.)

Blumhagen found that many patients felt they experienced a vicious circle whereby the social demands placed on them increased their blood pressure, and this in turn made them more stressed. Patients also gave credence to hereditary and physical factors such as obesity and excessive salt intake as being causes of their illness. Blumhagen constructed an elaborate model which attempted to bring together the complex causal sequences which patients described to him.

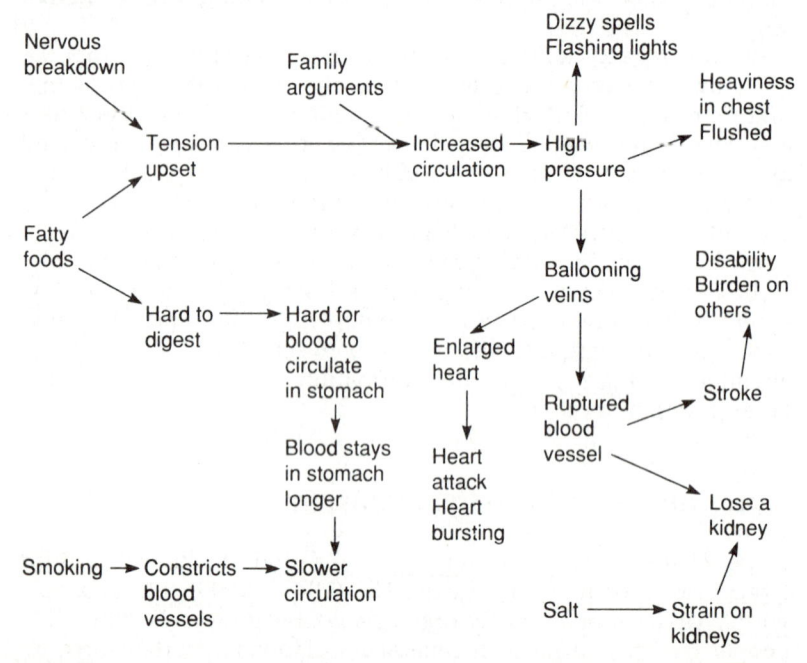

Fig. 4.1 An individual model of hypertension. (From Blumhagen, 1980. By permission of Kluwer Academic Publishers.)

Having interviewed the patients, Blumhagen also interviewed the nurse practitioners who treated them. They emphasized that the cause of hypertension was unknown, and they also expressed the view that it was made worse by stress. He developed a model based on the responses of the nurses which represented a more traditional expert view of hypertension which is shown on p. 31.

Our understanding of the patients' perspective was carried forward in Britain by Morgan and Watkins (1988) and Morgan (1993). They arranged for patients to be interviewed in general practice and compared the views of whites and Afro-Caribbeans living in London. They also found that stress was a popular explanation for hypertension. In addition, Morgan found that Afro-Caribbeans differed in their beliefs, and in their use of doctors and medical therapies. Afro-Caribbeans were more likely to report that they visited private doctors. One remarked:

Patients' ideas

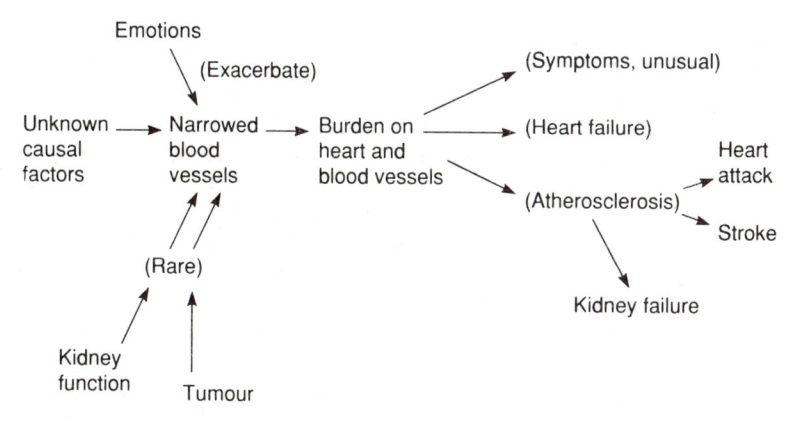

```
Emotions
    \ (Exacerbate)         ↗ (Symptoms, unusual)
Unknown → Narrowed → Burden on → (Heart failure)
causal    blood      heart and                      Heart
factors   vessels    blood vessels                ↗ attack
           ↑ ↑ ↑            ↘ (Atherosclerosis) →
          (Rare)                              ↘ Stroke
           ↑ ↑                    ↓
           │ │                Kidney failure
        Kidney │
        function Tumour
```

Fig. 4.2 A clinical model of hypertension. (From Blumhagen, 1980. By permission of Kluwer Academic Publishers.)

> 'It is no good going to a doctor and he starts to write a prescription out, like he is working in a factory – 'Next one, please.' – that sort of thing – off you go. No time available. Some of us realize this, so that's why we go and get another doctor'. (Morgan, 1993.)

The investigators found that more than half of the Afro-Caribbean patients used alternative remedies such as herbal tea. An advantage perceived by patients was that this treatment was natural and harmless. Afro-Caribbeans were much more concerned about the long-term effects of taking drugs. One said:

> 'No, I'd hate to think I have to keep taking tablets, but if I have to then I will end up a drug addict.' (Morgan, 1993.)

Another said:

> 'It bothers me taking the tablets long term because I don't know what the long term effects of the tablets will be. I don't think anybody does.' (Morgan, 1993.)

These concerns about dependency and future side effects were much more prevalent among Afro-Caribbean patients. In this context, it was common for them to 'leave off' the drugs on a semi-regular basis, taking the medication for only a few days each week. This practice was undertaken by both male and female patients.

Morgan and Watkins' (1988) work was qualitative. They aimed to uncover social meanings and processes from in-depth interviews with particular groups of people. Mhlongo (1992) used quantitative methods to test these associations on a larger group of patients. He sent a structured questionnaire to hypertensive patients in four practices, and 224 white and 203 Afro-Caribbean patients responded. He found that white patients were twice as likely to report that they were taking their medications as prescribed. One-third of Afro-Caribbean patients stated that they regularly took breaks from their medication or reduced the level. Afro-Caribbean patients were much more likely to use alternative remedies. They were also more likely to believe that they could recognize when their blood pressure was up because they experienced abnormal sensations in their head.

From these studies, it is possible to infer that patients' views of the causes of conditions and how they should be appropriately managed differ among different subcultural groups. Some of the views expressed may seem surprising to doctors. Moreover, the views reported may underestimate differences between doctors and patients. When told that they are hypertensive, those patients who differ most in their ideas from doctors may resist subsequent medicalization, and they may therefore not be included in studies of patients receiving therapy.

A group at McMaster University in Canada (Sackett et al., 1978; Taylor et al., 1981; MacDonald et al. 1984) looked at the effect of labelling men as hypertensive in an occupational setting. Two hundred and thirty hypertensive steel workers were identified and assessed with regard to their absenteeism the year before, and for 4 years after blood pressure screening had been undertaken. In the year prior to screening, men who were aware of their hypertension took on average almost twice as many days off for illness. In the 4 years following screening, absenteeism rose in the group who were newly identified as hypertensive. This occurred regardless of whether patients had been placed on medication or not. Patients who had been prescribed medication and did not comply with taking them showed an even larger rise in absenteeism from 2.6 days to 12 days per year. The investigators concluded that labelling a person as hypertensive may lead to a change in perception of his or her state of health, with the result that at least some patients were more ready to adopt the sick role when minor symptoms occurred.

Concern about the negative effect of labelling patients as hypertensive led researchers in Britain to study the emotional consequences of patients being told that their blood pressure was raised (Mann, 1981). During a national trial of the treatment of mild to moderate hypertension in general practice, a cohort of 235 consecutive trial entrants was studied by means of a psychiatric questionnaire and a standardized interview. Trial entrants were compared to a matched group of patients with normal blood pressure on screening, and with another cohort with raised blood pressure on screening which returned to normal without therapy. At the end of the follow-up year there was no difference in the incidence of psychiatric morbidity, and the prevalence of psychiatric morbidity actually fell among trial entrants. No measurement was made of absenteeism, as had been done in the Canadian study. Mann inferred that identifying the problem in general practice and providing regular follow-up support by practice nurses was advantageous in preventing negative psychological effects.

The results of these studies collectively suggest that health care providers may fail to offer maximal benefit, and may even do harm by identifying and labelling conditions without spending time with the patient on a continuing basis, encouraging them to express their ideas about the condition and its management.

An approach to remedying this deficit was developed by Inui *et al.* (1976). These physicians aimed to improve their effectiveness in managing patients with essential hypertension. A hospital outpatient clinic was identified where doctors acted as primary providers of health care for the local community and a third of the consultations were for hypertension. Initially, charts were reviewed and physicians were asked to estimate the percentage of time they spent taking a case history and examining the patient, and educating patients with respect to their hypertension and therapeutic regimens. Patients were interviewed in order to assess their knowledge and compliance with the drugs they were taking.

An educational intervention was then provided as a single tutorial session of 1–2 hours for half of the doctors. The teaching included the need for doctors to learn about their patients' ideas, and that discussion of this was important in achieving compliance with treatment and the prevention of complications. It was emphasized that learning about patients' ideas might be more important than the need for a traditional history and examination. The doctors also learned, from information gathered by the investigators, that their own patients were much less likely to be taking their pills than they had initially estimated.

Five months later, physicians were asked again to estimate the amount of time they spent on different activities during the consultation. Tutored doctors reported spending less time on taking a case history or undertaking physical examinations, and more time on reviewing medication and educating the patient. A review of the notes revealed more frequent entries by these doctors about patient compliance and understanding of the disease. The patients were subsequently visited at home. Patients who had seen doctors in the experimental group were almost twice as likely to be taking 75 per cent of their pills, and they knew significantly more about the complications of their condition. Blood pressure control in patients who had seen tutored physicians was also significantly better than that of the control group. The authors concluded that this form of educational intervention had the potential to improve patient compliance regarding medication and achieve better control of hypertension.

A stigmatized condition – epilepsy

Chronic conditions have continuing effects on patients in terms of their work, family life and self-management. Chronic neurological conditions are often particularly difficult for patients and doctors to understand and come to terms with. Problems affecting the brain are feared in society generally and possibly also by the medical profession. Despite the fact that neurological problems are exceedingly common, most doctors take a hands-off approach and leave the details of diagnosis and management to neurologists. In Britain, there are approximately six psychiatrists to every one neurologist, and each neurologist serves a population of about a quarter of a million people (Anon, 1994). With this ratio of specialists to patients, patients with chronic neurological conditions often receive inadequate information and advice. The care provided makes a travesty of the notion of a seamless service.

Scambler and Hopkins (1980, 1986), a sociologist and a neurologist respectively, decided to study the views of people with epilepsy. They identified 108 adults registered with 17 GPs, and 94 agreed to be interviewed by the investigators in their homes. The patients were all either taking drugs for epilepsy or had experienced one or more fits in the preceding 2 years. The investigators asked them about how the diagnosis had been made, about their work, driving and family relationships, and about their attitudes to their condition. They found that 48 per cent of patients had received their diagnosis from a specialist, whereas 36 per cent had been given the diagnosis by their GP. There was considerable uncertainty, and possibly denial, on both sides, with the result that almost half of the patients had learned about their diagnosis more than a year after their first attack. Most patients said they were upset, even resentful, when they were informed that they had epilepsy. The following interchange illustrates a typical response.

Interviewer: It was something about this word epilepsy that sparked that reaction off in you?

Patient: Mmn. Because, to me, when you tell people they sort of shun you, that's the way I look at it. They, you know, don't want to know; in fact my mother doesn't for one. If you go for a job and it's on a form – and you've got to put down 'yes' more often than not – you don't get the job, you know. (Scambler and Hopkins, 1986.)

Patients' negative perceptions about epilepsy and the uncertainty surrounding the diagnosis led many of them to try and negotiate for a less threatening label in the beginning. A few continued to deny or reject the diagnosis. The investigators found that 62 out of 94 of the subjects were ineligible to drive, but that despite this 12 of them were still doing so. Participation in work and disclosure of their condition were problematic issues for most epileptic patients. Only 42 were in full-time employment, and half of them had never disclosed their epilepsy at work. Only 11 patients had specifically informed their employers. Seven of them had informed their employers before starting work, two of whom did so because it was specified on the application form, and five because they suffered frequent seizures. Others told people at work only when the occurrence of a seizure made it necessary to do so.

Social relationships and the issue of disclosure were also difficult areas for people with epilepsy. Over 60 per cent of sufferers said they had never disclosed their condition to a boyfriend or girlfriend. A third disclosed the condition fully before marriage, but a third chose not to do so at all. Nearly 80 per cent of parents said they did not tell their children about their diagnosis! Patients described a sense of shame regardless of whether other people had actively discriminated against them or not. Ninety per cent of patients expressed this feeling, which the investigators called 'felt stigma'. But only one-third could recall actually being discriminated against; the investigators called this 'enacted stigma'. Scambler and Hopkins' account is an eye-opener for those who want to understand the patients' view about how it feels to live with questions of concealment and disclosure, and the feeling which the authors describe as having a 'spoiled identity'.

References

Anon (1994) Distinction awards: Analysis by type of award, speciality and percentage distribution at 31 December 1992, England and Wales. *Health Trends* 25: 1993–1994.

Blumhagen, D. (1980) Hyper-tension: A folk illness with a medical name. *Culture, Medicine and Psychiatry* 4: 197–227.

Campion, P. D. & Gabriel, J. (1985) Illness behaviour in mothers with young children. *Social Science and Medicine* 20: 325–330.

Cornford, C. S., Morgan, M. & Ridsdale, L. (1993) Why do mothers consult when their children cough? *Family Practice* 10: 193–196.

Inui, T., Yourtee, E. L. & Williamson, J. W. (1976) Improved outcomes in hypertension after physician tutorials. *Annals of Internal Medicine* 84: 646–651.

MacDonald, L. A., Sackett, D. L., Haynes, R. B. & Taylor, D. W. (1984) Labelling in hypertension: A review of the behavioral and psychological consequences. *Journal of Chronic Disease* 37: 933–942.

Mann, A. H. (1981) Factors affecting psychological states during one year on a hypertension trial. *Clinical and Investigative Medicine* 4: 197–200.

Mhlongo, S. (1992) *Hypertension: Lay Beliefs and Responses Concerning Hypertension and its Management in Two Culturally Distinct Groups.* UMDS Department of General Practice, London: MSc dissertation.

Morgan, M. (1993) *Beliefs and Responses to Hypertension: Patients and Practitioners' Perspectives.* London: University of London PhD.

Morgan, M. & Watkins, C. J. (1988) Managing hypertension: Beliefs and responses to medication among cultural groups. *Sociology of Health and Illness* 10: 561–578.

Office of Population Consenses and Surveys (1993) *Mortality Statistics: Cause 1992.* Series DH2 (19). London: HMSO.

Royal College of General Practitioners, Office of Population Censuses and Surveys, and Department of Health (1986) *Morbidity Statistics from General Practice. Third National Study, 1981–1982.* London: HMSO.

Sackett, D. L., Haynes, R. B., Taylor, D. W., Gibson, E. S. & Johnson, A. L. (1978) Increased absenteeism from work after detection and labelling of hypertensive patients. *New England Journal of Medicine* 299: 741–744.

Scambler, G. & Hopkins, A. (1980) Social class, epileptic activity, and disadvantage at work. *Journal of Epidemiology and Community Health* 34: 129–133.

Scambler, G. & Hopkins, A. (1986) Being epileptic – coming to terms with stigma. *Sociology of Health and Illness* 8: 26–43.

Taylor, D. W., Haynes, R. B., Sackett, D. L. & Gibson, E. S. (1981) Long term follow-up of absenteeism among working men following the detection and treatment of their hypertension. *Clinical and Investigative Medicine* 4: 173–177.

5
Psychological Distress in General Practice

> Mrs Yardley comes in and bursts into tears. She says her husband has told her he has found someone else ....

> Mr and Mrs Chard come together. He has rapidly lost weight with a pancreatic cancer. The problem has been explained to him, but he is still asking for reassurance that he will get better. His wife says he is very angry and irritable with her, and asks if she can see a counsellor.

> A trainer identifies 20 per cent of her patients as having emotional problems. The trainee finds 10 per cent of the patients who visit him have emotional problems. How can this be explained?

How much of it is there?

I have chosen as my starting point the assumption that emotional distress is as easy to define and measure as warts or chicken pox. This assumption will be challenged subsequently and the complex issues discussed in stages. Emotional distress is common in the community, and according to psychiatrists approximately 20 per cent (Williams et al., 1986) of the population suffer from it at any given point in time. Many individuals affected by it will not go to see their doctors. Some may not recognize that they have a problem, some may obtain adequate support from family and friends, and some may think that their problems cannot be solved by medical personnel. But in one practice, over a third of patients reported that when they did have an emotional problem they had confided this to their general practitioner (Corney, 1990a). It is to be expected, therefore, that patients visiting the surgery will report more symptoms of emotional distress than those in the community at large. Goldberg and Bridges (1987) found one-third of attenders reported having emotional problems when asked. Once in the surgery, patients vary in their choice of the doctor to whom they wish to divulge emotional problems, and doctors vary with regard to the asking of psychosocial questions and the number of cases they identify.

Most problems go no further than this and are not medicalized. A very small proportion of patients identified as having psychological problems are referred to psychiatrists. And psychiatrists decide to treat only a small and decreasing proportion of those referred in hospital.

Bearing this process in mind, the psychiatric morbidity which is identified as such depends on decision-making by patients, GPs and in a few cases by psychiatrists. The severity of illness does increase along the path from GP to psychiatrist, with in-patients being far more likely to have psychotic problems compared to the emotional distress which is common in general practice.

Who gets it?

The answer to this question is not as straightforward as it seems. It depends to a certain extent on who is most likely to acknowledge psychological symptoms, who GPs identify as having problems and the extent to which GPs are able to recognize symptoms. Patients who say that they are unemployed are more likely to be diagnosed as having psychiatric problems, as are those who finished their education earlier, which is often found to be the case among those in lower socio-economic groups (Boardman, 1987). Those who are married but living apart are recognized as having more psychiatric morbidity than their married or single counterparts, and single men are described as having more psychiatric morbidity than their married contemporaries.

What forms do GPs see?

Many of the psychological problems patients present to GPs are problems such as anxiety and depression. Some of these are associated with physical illness. Physical symptoms frequently provide an 'entry ticket' for patients with underlying depression or anxiety. The two cases described at the beginning of the chapter illustrate typical presentations. Weighing up physical, psychological and social components is a major task for the general practitioner.

A small minority of attenders have more severe psychological impairments like schizophrenia or manic depressive illness. Doctors vividly remember the times when they have had to arrange an acute admission for these patients. A third major group of patients GPs see or hear about from others in the community have fixed or maladaptive patterns of relating, including complaining and dependant individuals. These individuals with 'personality disorders' cause their families and doctors continuing heartache as there appear to be few solutions to their ongoing problems.

Why do GPs miss cases?

Doctor factors

The ability of GPs to identify psychological distress in their patients varies a great deal. This has been demonstrated in research experiments (Jenkins et al., 1988), by psychiatrists visiting general practices (Marks et al., 1979), and by examining the diagnoses recorded by GPs in the general practice morbidity survey (Dunn and Smeeton, 1989).

This variation suggests that GPs practise psychological medicine in a subjective and idiosyncratic way. Why is this so? Firstly, all GPs have undergone only a few months training in psychiatry as undergraduates, and some have done another six months or so at postgraduate level. This training may have focused on the small minority of patients with severe, often psychotic disease who are admitted to psychiatric hospitals. Knowledge and skills about how to identify and manage the sorts of psychological problems more frequently seen in the community is largely acquired in general practice. Secondly, Howie and colleagues (1991) have demonstrated that psychosocial problems are more often identified during longer consultations. The remuneration of British GPs provides an incentive to look after more patients, but not to spend more time with each of them. In some countries, for example Canada, doctors can claim extra fees for time spent with patients with psychosocial problems. In view of the incentive structure in Britain, it is not surprising, as Calnan (1988) demonstrated, that those doctors who are financially oriented express less interest in patients with psychosocial problems.

Patient factors

Of the cases described, GPs are likely to find it easier to identify the first patient who came in, burst into tears and said her husband wanted to leave her as suffering from psychological distress. Other patients are more difficult to identify and classify, given that general practitioners may be short of time. Freeling *et al.* (1985) showed that GPs particularly tend to overlook depression in patients with a co-existing physical illness. In the brief time span of the consultation, doctors may understandably focus on identifying and managing the physical symptoms. Doctors may also regard emotional distress as a normal consequence of loss of health and well-being.

Goldberg and Bridges (1987) found that GPs also overlook psychological disorders when patients present with physical symptoms. General practitioners may in some cases first decide to investigate possible physical causes, but in doing this they may inadvertently medicalize patients who somatize. This is a challenge for physicians generally. For some patients, investigations which yield normal results are reassuring. For others, tests may foster the conviction that they do have an organic disease. The system of remuneration on a capitation basis for this kind of problem has the advantage that the GP can negotiate with the patient about his or her conceptions over a long period. Patients in the British private sector or other fee for service systems may leave the doctor who will not search for an organic cause and does not have the time to negotiate, and shop around in search of more investigations.

'Scientific factors'

The patient's characteristics, the doctor's training and attitudes, and economic incentives have all been identified as factors contributing to GPs missing 'cases'. But at least some of the blame can legitimately be placed on confusion within the area of psychiatry about what mental illness is and how it can be measured. A research psychiatrist (Birchnell, 1974) has suggested that 'there is no observable or measurable representation of mental illness so its presence is largely a matter of the psychiatrist's opinion'.

Part of the training in any specialty involves learning to report observations in an agreed way. Without physical landmarks, it is difficult for psychiatrists to agree on symptoms and therefore report on a diagnosis in a standardized way. Psychiatrists vary a great deal in their diagnoses too. In one study, Kreitman and coworkers (1961) found psychiatrists agreed on making a generic diagnosis of neurosis 52 per cent of the time. But they agreed on the specific category of neurosis, for example depressive neurosis, only

28 per cent of the time. Lack of training or time cannot explain this variation. Relating the psychological symptoms expressed by patients to diagnostic labels is difficult for everyone.

Ideal types

The diagnosis of psychiatric problems in general practice depends on the models that are available in science and in society which inform patients' and doctors' decision-making. Diagnostic probabilities may also have a self-fulfilling quality. Women, for example, are more likely to identify their symptoms as emotional and to take them to doctors. And doctors perceive more psychiatric illness in female patients than male patients independently of the patients' symptomatology (Marks et al., 1979). Doctors are more likely to identify a psychiatric disorder in known high-risk groups such as people who are married but living apart, the unemployed and those who left school earlier. And when individuals experience emotional problems and are in 'low-risk' groups such as educated men in full-time employment, their problems are less likely to be identified by their doctor (Boardman, 1987). This problem of self-fulfilling expectations is not unique to psychiatry. However, because the 'signs' of psychiatric illness are verbal and relatively intangible, it is particularly difficult to measure illness objectively in this area.

What is psychiatric illness?

Having initially assumed that psychiatry in general practice is well defined, we need to ask: what is a case of psychiatric illness? Research psychiatrists are prone to answer this question with another question: for what purpose are you seeking to know? Epidemiologists are interested in knowing how much of it there is about. General practitioners are more interested in knowing the answers to different questions like: how do you identify what is treatable, and what is identifiable but not time-effective to treat? This raises additional questions about the natural history of psychiatric illness with and without treatment. These pragmatic but fundamental questions will be discussed below.

Research psychiatrists have developed structured interviews in an effort to standardize the way in which psychiatric cases are diagnosed. The Clinical Interview Schedule (Goldberg and Blackwell, 1970) and the Present State Examination (Wing et al., 1981), both developed at the Institute of Psychiatry, are most often used by researchers in Britain. A research psychiatrist working in the community or in general practice might spend an hour or more with each person asking him or her a standard set of questions with supplementary questions if answers to stem questions are positive. The investigator would then be able to collate data about symptoms, severity and timing and classify the patient's problems. A clinician trained to use the same instrument should be able to repeat the process and achieve similar results. This is the 'gold standard' used by researchers.

It would not be cost-effective for GPs to spend an hour or more with each patient in order to identify psychiatric cases reliably. Psychiatrists have developed shorter screening methods to identify likely cases in general practice. Two well validated examples are the General Health Questionnaire (GHQ) (Goldberg and Williams, 1988) and the Hospital Anxiety and Depression Scale (Zigmond and Snaith, 1983), which are both lists of symptoms that patients can read and endorse. The more symptoms that the patient acknowledges having on the checklist, the more he or she is likely to be suffering from psychological distress. It is a non-specific test, rather like measuring the erythrocyte sedimentation rate. The choice of cut-off point at which it is likely that the patient has a disorder is arbitrary.

Research psychiatrists and GPs have used the GHQ to measure the prevalence of patients presenting to GPs with a particular number of psychological symptoms, and compared the result with the identification by GPs of those symptoms. Depending on the cut-off point used, GPs failed to identify between a quarter and a third of patients who acknowledge symptoms of emotional distress on a self-administered questionnaire (Goldberg and Williams, 1988). GPs wishing to improve their ability to identify psychological problems can compare the results of questionnaires like this one with their own performance as a learning technique.

What causes the psychological distress presented in general practice?

Causes of psychiatric morbidity seen in general practice have been actively investigated during the past 20 years. The conventional psychiatric wisdom in Britain was that depression was reactive in some cases and endogenous in others. The sociologists Brown and Harris (1978) postulated that depression might generally be the consequence of adverse life events and difficulties, in the context of relatively weak social support mechanisms. This research hypothesis fits well with general practitioners' personal and experiential knowledge.

Brown and Harris (1978) chose to focus on working class women, as their depression rates were particularly high. From their work, they inferred that women at home with young children were particularly vulnerable when stressful life events occurred, and they postulated that an intimate and confiding relationship protected women from depression. This proposition was supported by evidence derived retrospectively. Brown et al. (1986) subsequently retested this association using a prospective design. Using a two-stage method, the investigators assessed the support given by close ties before and after stressful events occurred. A close tie was defined as a husband, lover or someone named as very close at first contact.

An intimate and confiding relationship had been defined after the events described in the first study, and it was associated with a protective effect when stressful life events occurred. However, in the prospective study an intimate and confiding relationship was defined at the start. When these relationships were tested and withstood life events there was a reduced risk of the woman developing clinical depression. But of married women who were receiving support at the start of the study, 40 per cent did not receive support at the time of a crisis in the follow-up year. Women let down by not receiving the support they expected had a particularly high rate of depression.

This illustrates how difficult it is to measure social phenomena, such as life events and social support. It is important to apply different research designs to test a hypothesis, and a prospective study is superior to a retrospective one. Although social research like this is difficult, the results seem to match the experience of doctors working in the community.

What is the natural history or outcome of the psychiatric morbidity seen in general practice?

This is an important question for general practitioners in Britain, where in contrast to promotion and preventive activities which are highly remunerated, there is no financial incentive to identify and treat psychological problems. Jenkins and co-workers (1981) undertook a prospective study to follow up patients for 1 year after the GP identified a psychological problem. They interviewed patients using the Clinical Interview Schedule, and in addition developed a structured social interview in which they enquired about occupation, finance, housing, social relationships, marriage and family.

One hundred patients were admitted to the study. Seventy-two were women, many of whom were housewives. At the end of the study year, the investigators found that approximately 50 per cent of patients had recovered. A specific psychiatric diagnosis was not helpful in predicting outcome, but the severity rating of the psychiatric disorder was. The rating given on the basis of a social interview was more useful in predicting outcome; a supportive family life was associated with improvement in the follow-up year, whereas a stressful family life was associated with a chronic pattern of illness. This suggests that it is more helpful prognostically for GPs to enquire about the social factors that predispose individuals to psychological dysfunction than to categorize the psychological disorder *per se*.

When studying the epidemiology of most diseases, it is assumed that morbidity and mortality are related as measures of outcome in the natural history of disease. In psychiatric illness this is not necessarily so. For example, it is sometimes assumed that in treating the most common affective disorder, depression, the final measure of outcome might be prevention of death by suicide. But the social characteristics of those who present with depression and those who successfully suicide are not the same. This suggests that they are not necessarily different stages on a continuum.

Women are two to three times more likely to be classified as depressed than men, and this is particularly true of the lower socio-economic classes. Men are three times as likely as women to die from suicide (OPCS, 1993), and the incidence of suicide is relatively high in socio-economic groups like doctors. These trends suggest that identifying and treating depression and other minor psychiatric morbidity in general practice may have little impact on death rates through suicide. The natural history of minor psychiatric morbidity is that some illnesses resolve completely, some resolve and relapse, and some are chronic.

Does identification make any difference?

Most research in general practice has focused on identifying psychiatric morbidity. However, there would not be much point in doing this unless it could be demonstrated that identification led to increased benefits or reduced harms.

Corney (1990b) reviewed the literature on counselling in general practice and found that there was little hard evidence that counselling either by general practitioners or by counsellors improved the outcome of patients with psychological problems. She found more evidence that counselling by nurses and social workers had demonstrable benefits. There are problems with the studies done so far. Firstly, it is likely that counselling benefits some conditions more than others, and these first need to be identified. Secondly, the packages offered as counselling by general practitioners and counsellors probably vary considerably in style, quantity and quality. Until standardized training is provided for professionals, and packages are developed for targeted conditions, it will be difficult to confirm what is truly beneficial.

A second therapeutic option is to treat patients with drugs. The demonstrated harms of chronic benzodiazepine use have led to a reduction in GP prescribing of these drugs. But antidepressants do seem to work. Hollyman *et al.* (1988) undertook a double-blind placebo controlled trial of amitryptyline for depressed patients in general practice. At the time of their study, some general practitioners avoided drug therapy or used antidepressants at subtherapeutic doses. Ninety patients were admitted to the study and given amitryptyline, while 88 patients were in the placebo group. Twenty-three patients in the treatment group and 14 patients in the placebo group failed to complete 4 weeks' treatment. Follow-up using research interviews and questionnaires showed that those who had continued to take their drugs at 4 weeks were significantly improved compared to the placebo treated group.

Ideally, the mental state of all the patients admitted to the study would have been reported, including those who failed to complete their treatment who were in the 'intention to treat group'. Nevertheless, these results do support the notion that patients who are prescribed an antidepressant in therapeutic doses and take them will benefit in terms of their psychiatric state. Presumably, the patients who experienced on balance more adverse effects than benefits from the medication withdrew from treatment. This is an important study and it deserves to be replicated if GPs are to be convinced of the value of prescribing antidepressants in therapeutic doses.

A third specific option is referral, particularly for anxiety or phobias, to a psychologist or psychiatric nurse for cognitive therapy. The benefits of these therapies have been demonstrated (Marks, 1985; Ross and Scott, 1985). Direct access to psychologists and psychiatric nurses makes this an increasingly useful option.

Should GPs screen patients for psychological problems?

Does screening by questionnaire, and identifying patients who would not otherwise be identified, result in treatment that reduces the severity or duration of emotional distress? Johnstone and Goldberg (1976) undertook a controlled trial in which patients filled in a questionnaire, the results of which were made available to the GP on a randomized basis. The investigators reported that when the GP was made aware of the reported symptoms through the GHQ, the duration and severity of symptoms was reduced in the ensuing year.

The prospective randomized design of this study was ahead of its time, but assessments of outcome were undertaken in a non-blind way by the GP who had been responsible for therapy. It is not clear whether this introduced observer bias which accounted for the reported difference between the experimental and control groups. Subsequent studies have failed to reproduce the beneficial outcome. Those who urge GPs to screen patients with psychiatric symptoms using questionnaires must demonstrate that there is a difference in outcome before GPs start using instruments like this in everyday practice as opposed to learning situations.

Labelling – good or bad?

It could be argued that labelling *per se* prevents harms, even though it is of no direct therapeutic benefit. For example, GPs sometimes express the belief that identifying the depression which underlies the presentation of somatic symptoms may prevent a patient being sent for unnecessary, expensive and potentially harmful investigations. It is difficult to test this hypothesis with research, so this must remain a belief.

Secondly, if the GP identifies a psychological problem which is likely to be chronic, for example, a personality disorder, he or she will be able to consider the relative costs of spending more time with this patient, rather than with a patient who has a problem for which treatment has been demonstrated to have a beneficial effect, such as depression. Trainees and young doctors sometimes unrealistically believe they can be successful in helping a patient improve where others have failed. Anecdotally, those who leave general practice seem to report disillusion and burn out, and perhaps part of this was due to spending too much time and energy with patients who did not change. This is a difficult topic for research, but identifying psychiatric disorders accurately may prevent harm for both patients and doctors.

Labelling may also have negative effects for patients. Illich (1976) and Foucault (1981) have attacked the use of obscure and alienating language by the medical profession. Illich (1976) wrote that when 'language is taken over by the doctors, the sick person is deprived of meaningful words for this anguish which is thus further increased by linguistic mystification'. Foucault argued that the medical profession has taken over the priest's role in advising families and imposing its own labels, which increase the mystique of the profession without necessarily helping patients.

It is difficult to test these theories, which form a major critique of society and the role of the professions. There is some evidence that patients may want to be listened to, but not necessarily categorized, when they experience psychological distress. Boardman (1987) measured psychological distress in male and female patients consulting GPs in South London. He found that patients with higher scores on the GHQ, and particularly male patients, were more likely to consult female partners in the practices. These doctors were less likely to label problems as 'psychological'.

It may be that Illich and Foucault are right. Patients may want to talk about the life events and difficulties they experience without being labelled and pathologized. They may choose women doctors, believing they are more likely to listen without necessarily labelling them. This is speculation, and more work needs to be done to explore what is going on. As patients increasingly gain access to their notes, it is important that GPs continue to debate and investigate the benefits and harms of naming and intervening when psychosocial problems are presented to them. A tactic used by American doctors when presented by patients experiencing life events and difficulties is to use the diagnosis 'transient situational disturbance'. This social category, derived from the American Psychiatric Association (1987), recommends itself as a non-pejorative label which might be applied to many of the psychosocial problems brought to the GP.

References

American Psychiatric Association (1987) *Diagnostic and Statistical Manual of Mental Disorders DSM-III-R.* Washington: American Psychiatric Association.

Birchnell, J. (1974) Is there a scientifically acceptable alternative to the epidemiological study of familial factors in mental illness? *Social Science and Medicine 8:* 335–350.

Boardman, J. (1987) The General Health Questionnaire and the detection of emotional disorders by general practitioners. *British Journal of Psychiatry 151:* 373–381.

Brown, G. W. & Harris, T. O. (1978) *Social Origins of Depression.* Andover: Tavistock Publications.

Brown, G. W., Andrews, B., Harris, T., Adler, Z. & Bridge, L. (1986) Social support, self-esteem and depression. *Psychological Medicine 16:* 813–31.

Calnan, M. (1988) Images of general practice: The perceptions of the doctor. *Social Science and Medicine 27:* 579–586.

Corney, R. H. (1990a) A survey of professional help sought by patients with psychosocial problems. *British Journal of General Practice 40:* 365–368.

Corney, R. H. (1990b) Counselling in general practice – does it work? Discussion paper. *Journal of the Royal Society of Medicine 83:* 253–257.

Dunn, G. & Smeeton, N. (1989) The study of episodes of psychiatric morbidity. In: P. Williams, G. Wilkinson & K. Rawnsley (eds) *The Scope of Epidemiological Psychiatry.* London: Routledge.

Foucault, M. (1981) *The History of Sexuality.* Middlesex: Pelican Books.

Freeling, P., Rao, B. M., Paykel, E. S., Sireling, L. I. & Burton, R. H. (1985) Unrecognised depression in general practice. *British Medical Journal 29:* 1880–1883.

Goldberg, D. P. & Blackwell, B. (1970) Psychiatric illness in general practice. A detailed study using a new method of case identification. *British Medical Journal* 2: 439–443.

Goldberg, D. P. & Bridges, K. (1987) Screening for psychiatric illness in general practice: The general practitioners versus the screening questionnaire. *Journal of the Royal College of General Practitioners* 43: 15–18.

Goldberg, D. & Williams, P. (1988) *A User's Guide to the General Health Questionnaire (GHQ)*. Windsor: NFER–Nelson Publishing Co.

Hollyman, J. A., Freeling, P., Paykel, E. S., Bhat, A. & Sedgwick, P. (1988) Double-blind placebo-controlled trial of amitryptyline among depressed patients in general practice. *Journal of the Royal College of General Practitioners* 38: 393–397.

Howie, J. G. R., Porter, A. M. D., Heaney, D. J. & Hopton, J. L. (1991) Long to short consultation ratio: A proxy measure of quality of care for general practice. *British Journal of General Practice* 41: 48–54.

Illich, I. (1976) *Limits to Medicine*. Middlesex: Penguin Books.

Jenkins, R., Mann, A. H. & Belsey, E. (1981) The background, design and use of short interview to assess social stress and support in research and clinical settings. *Social Science and Medicine* 15: 195–203.

Jenkins, R., Smeeton, N. & Shepherd, M. (1988) Classification of mental disorder in primary care. *Psychological Medicine*, Monograph Supplement no. 12.

Johnstone, A. & Goldberg, D. (1976) Psychiatric screening in general practice: A controlled trial. *The Lancet* i: 605–608.

Kreitman, N., Sainsbury, P., Morrissey, J., Towers, J. & Scrivenor, J. (1961) The reliability of psychiatric assessment: An analysis. *Journal of Mental Science* 107: 887–908.

Marks, I. (1985) Controlled trial of psychiatric nurse therapists in primary care. *British Medical Journal* 290: 1181–1184.

Marks, J. N., Goldberg, D. P. & Hillier, V. F. (1979) Determinants of the ability of general practitioners to detect psychiatric illness. *Psychological Medicine* 9: 337–353.

Office of Population Censuses and Surveys (1993) *Mortality Statistics: Cause 1992*. Series DH2 (19). London: HMSO.

Ross, M. & Scott, M. (1985) An evaluation of the effectiveness of individual and group cognitive therapy in the treatment of depressed patients in an inner city health centre. *Journal of the Royal College of General Practitioners* 35: 239–242.

Williams, P., Tarnspolsky, A., Hand, D. & Shepherd, M. (1986) Minor psychiatric morbidity and general practice consultation. Psychological Medicine, Monograph Supplement No. 9.

Wing, J. K., Bebbington, P. & Robbins, L. N. (1981) *What is a Case – The Problem of Definition in Psychiatric Community Surveys*. London: Grant McIntyre.

Zigmond, A. & Snaith, R. (1983) The Hospital Anxiety and Depression Scale. *Acta Psychiatrica Scandinavica* 67: 361–70.

RCGP Examination Question

Discuss the evidence concerning the detection and management of depression in general practice. Critical Reading Paper, 5 May 1993.

6

Communication During the Consultation

Consultation models

Balint's biographical approach

Balint (1957), a psychoanalyst, developed an international reputation for encouraging GPs to work in groups and review their difficult patients. The GPs described their patients, many of whom were unhappy women coming to the doctor with physical complaints. Some of them were, to use current technical language, somatizers. Balint's teaching was to look beyond the physical 'ticket of entry', and search for meaning in the patient's terms.

Instead of the pharmaceutical remedies, like Valium, frequently prescribed during that period, Balint encouraged doctors to offer more of themselves, and implicitly more of their time and empathy. He also drew attention to the difference between the doctors' and the patients' view of appropriate consulting behaviour. Balint's quasi-religious term, 'the apostolic function' (1957) seems to describe the doctor's mission to teach and convert patients to their own beliefs about what it is appropriate to consult the doctor with. This mission ran counter to themes developing in sociology and medical ethics concerning lay beliefs, illness behaviour and patients' autonomy. Balint did not value doctors taking up fixed positions. He pioneered a practice by which doctors, often by analyzing their conflicts with patients, make small but significant changes which involve personal growth.

Byrne and Long's phases and styles

Byrne and Long's work (1976) included the creation of new models, measurement and evaluation of a teaching intervention. Their model involved six phases:
   1. Relating.
   2. Discovering the reason for attendance.

3. A verbal or physical examination, or both.
4. Consideration of the condition.
5. Advising on treatment.
6. Terminating the interview.

The cognitive structure of 'phases' helped doctors to appraise what was and what was not achieved.

Byrne and Long also introduced the concept of a spectrum of consultations which ranged from those which were 'doctor-centred' to those which were 'patient-centred', and they developed a set of criteria to measure these qualities. It then became all too easy for some doctors to apply these terms without applying the instruments Byrne and Long had used to measure consulting behaviour. These doctors assumed that the desire or attempt to improve was synonymous with achieving 'patient-centred' consultations. 'Patient-centred' medicine became a shibboleth in general practice. Teachers and trainees used the term as though it were self-revealing, without mentioning the need for measurement. It was a means by which some doctors attributed good or bad labels to others which was potentially self-deluding and divisive.

Widening the agenda

Stott and Davis (1979) set out their potential agenda for the consultation. Like Balint, they drew attention to the need to consider and modify patients' ideas about appropriate consulting behaviour. Additionally, they prioritized two other components: dealing with health promotion and continuing problems. The 1990 contract and desktop data processing have simultaneously increased these tasks and facilitated their completion.

Pull skills

Pendleton and his colleagues (1984) not only adopted a well orchestrated approach, but also one which came at just the right moment. Their approach enabled doctors to respond to research done by psychologists, anthropologists and sociologists on patients' cognitions and lay beliefs. These were described in Chapter 4. Qualitative research had focused on the elaborate explanations and personal knowledge that patients, families and subcultures develop about the cause of their diseases and their appropriate management. The evidence from this research helped to justify doctors' need for advanced communication skills, if they wished to advise and change the behaviour of people in the community. The adequacy of techniques for taking case histories and communication skills as learned in the hospital setting had been called into question. This lacuna in the field of communication skills was demonstrated by a psychologist, Roter (1977). She taught hospital outpatients to be more active and questioning, but no change was introduced into the doctors' skills. The result was that after their consultations this group of patients became more anxious, angry and dissatisfied than a comparison group.

Pendleton and his colleagues (1984) emphasized that doctors needed a communication template with which they could search out patients' ideas, concerns and expectations, and use them to achieve a negotiated agreement. This dynamic model of negotiation fitted ethical principles concerning informed consent and autonomous decision-making by patients. This new approach to the consultation was rapidly disseminated among young doctors, partially as a result of close co-operation between the psychologist, Pendleton and some general practitioners in producing and providing an educational package. An obstacle to progress initially was the lack of reliable and valid instruments to measure progress in applying the technique, and quantitative research based on this.

A human development approach

Neighbour (1987) defined five consultation tasks or phases.
 1. Connecting with the patient.
 2. Summarizing the problem.
 3. Handing over responsibility for management.
 4. Safety-netting.
 5. Housekeeping.

The first three tasks emerged from earlier work. The final two tasks added new and important emphases and will be described in more detail. After sharing ideas about, for example, a child's stomach pain, the doctor needs to 'safety-net'. This involves explaining to the carer other possible causes of the pain, and how future characteristics such as its duration and severity might change the ordering of diagnostic probabilities. This sharing of knowledge, uncertainty and the responsibility for decision-making involves a synthesis of medical ethics, problem-solving and communication.

'Housekeeping' was the final task. Neighbour explained that doctors need to sustain their own mental and physical energy and awareness throughout the consulting process. Howie *et al.* (1991) subsequently demonstrated that heavily booked surgeries were associated with declining performance measurements. It is likely that without proper attention to the scheduling of appointments and rests, doctor fatigue regularly leads to declining and suboptimal performance during the working day.

Neighbour emphasized Maslow's (1970) model which suggested that all humans (including doctors) need rest and an opportunity for self-expression in order to function well. Doctors who believe and act as though they do not have these needs risk reducing the meeting of two humans to a mechanical assembly line process, which is insensitive and alienating for their patients. This task of self-care is extremely difficult to achieve on a day-to-day basis in a profession which traditionally identified itself with a macho work ethos, and a contract specifying continuous service to others. Aspects of personal growth are also difficult to achieve and difficult to measure except in an individual, inter-subjective way. But they are important and deserve more research in future.

Measurement of process and outcome

A self-audit

The current fashion for audit involves a pre-measurement guess at what an acceptable standard might be. This first guess may deter some GPs, because they fear they will not live up to their own stated ideals. Others participate in an audit, and are then disappointed when they find that in measuring their activities they have fallen short of their own targets. This sense of disappointment can be especially painful when measuring performance in the consulting room, where doctors particularly want to believe that their behaviour conforms to whatever they consider to be 'good', for example, being patient-centred. This is perhaps one reason why there has been so little measurement of the consultation process.

Bain (1976) designed an instrument to measure statements made during his own tape-recorded consultations. An advantage of his method was that it did not require pre-measurement target setting. It was simple to apply and learn from in an inductive way. The statements he identified and measured were social exchange, facilitation, questions asked by the doctor and patients, and explanations by the doctor of the problem and its management. Using these categories of statements, Bain learned inductively about what he actually did. He found that he talked at least as much as the patient. He also found that on average he talked and listened more to middle class than to working class patients.

He was able to construct a histogram to show the distribution of statements in the consultation. This consisted of two main parts which can be defined as:
1. getting information (or 'pull') behaviours, for example, questions and facilitation, which he used in the first half of the consultation,
2. and giving information (or 'push') behaviours, with which the doctor provided information and explained his decision-making in the second half of the consultation.

By analyzing the data further, Bain found that middle class patients were more verbally active, using their own verbal (pull) skills more to question the doctor and express their own ideas.

Dysfunctional consultations

Byrne and Long (1976) formulated a model of what should happen during the consultation. Having done this, they measured what occurred in GPs' consultations using their own set of criteria and research instruments. They were particularly interested in what makes consultations go wrong. The investigators found that consultations which went wrong were more likely to take place in the evening and were shorter on average. More butting in and less silence occurred. Less time was spent on the second phase of the consultation, when the doctor should have found out why the patient had come. If this was cut short, the investigators inferred that the doctor ran the risk of making assumptions about the patient which were not necessarily shared by the patient him or herself.

GPs as poor 'pullers' and negotiators

Tuckett and his colleagues' (1985) theory of how doctors should consult with patients was based on the sociological evidence previously described, that patients have complex ideas about the cause of disease. It was also based on the ethical principle that patients need information in order to decide themselves what is best for them. Their model of the autonomous patient who is an expert on his or her own health is particularly relevant when considering the extent to which health education information provided by doctors is taken up by patients.

The investigators used sophisticated methods to evaluate doctors' consultation skills and interviewed patients at length in their homes to assess their reactions to the doctors' advice and their intention to comply with the advice given. The researchers reported that the doctors they studied did not generally manage to achieve a dialogue or share and exchange views with patients. Whereas doctors spent time explaining their own views, they did little to encourage patients to present their views. The investigators also found that doctors frequently actively inhibited patients from asking questions, or evaded answering patients' questions. This occurred two to three times more frequently when doctors dealt with women patients. Doctors rarely explored whether a patient understood what they said, and doctors did not usually tailor advice and instructions to known details of the patient's life.

When Tuckett and his co-workers (1985) interviewed the patients after their consultations, the investigators did find a relationship between the quality of advice and communication in the consultation and the short-term outcome, in terms of patients' stated evaluation of and commitment to the doctors' advice. The investigators found that in consultations where there was evidence that a doctor had inhibited or evaded a patient's ideas, patients were less likely to be committed to the doctor's advice. They also found that women, women bringing children, younger patients and those from ethnic minorities were least likely to be committed to the doctor's ideas about the diagnosis. Women presenting babies under 2 years and ethnic minority groups were also least likely to be committed to the doctor's treatment plan.

These findings suggest that doctors are not necessarily good communicators or health educationalists, and they are not good at applying the models of Pendleton. One explanation for Tuckett *et al.*'s findings is that most of the GPs started practising before vocational training began and may have had no specific training in how to share ideas, facilitate learning and influence decision-making by patients. Average talking time during the consultation was 7 minutes, with 1 minute for the examination. This time was much shorter than that available to the social scientists who interviewed patients in their homes without the competing pressures of differential diagnoses. Nonetheless, Tuckett's work can be seen as a challenge to the truism that GPs are 'patient-centred', or that GPs are necessarily experts in communication.

Doctors' skills and outcomes

North American investigators have done more work on relating the process of communication to the outcome. Francis and colleagues (1969) studied consultations in which mothers brought their children to physicians. They tape-recorded consultations and carried out follow-up interviews 7–14 days later, to assess satisfaction and compliance in terms of advice taken and medication. The investigators found that the mothers who expected to have an explanation of the nature and cause of their child's illness, and who failed to receive this explanation, were less likely to be satisfied or to comply with the advice given. They were also less likely to comply if the doctor did not seem to understand their concerns.

Satisfaction with the consultation overall was significantly related to compliance. The investigators inferred that doctors' ability to influence their patients' health related behaviour depended on their skills as communicators. Although outcome research is difficult, more evidence of this kind is needed before sceptics as well as 'true believers' spend more time and energy on learning and practising their listening and explaining skills.

In Canada, Henbest and Stewart (1990) have developed an instrument to measure what they call 'patient-centredness' in audiotaped consultations. They defined 'patient-centredness' as care in which the doctor responded to the patient in such a way as to allow the patient to express his or her reasons for coming to the doctor, including symptoms, expectations, thoughts and feelings. After the consultation, patients were interviewed and a telephone interview was carried out 2 weeks later. This could be a way to measure the desirable behaviours described by Pendleton and his colleagues (1984).

The investigators found that patients who had received the highest level of patient-centred responses to their main symptom were significantly more likely to have decreased concern about that symptom immediately after their consultation than patients who had experienced fewer patient-centred responses. At 2 weeks, however, there was no significant association between patient-centred responses and symptom resolution. This study was important for the development of a new measure and deserves to be repeated with larger numbers.

Patients' skills and outcomes

Most research on communication during the consultation has started from the premiss that doctors need to change to produce improved outcome. A novel approach of working with patients to improve their assertiveness was adopted by Roter (1977) and developed further by Kaplan (in Stewart and Roter, 1989) and Greenfield et al. (1988). They trained an experimental group of patients with diabetes and hypertension to be more assertive and use their negotiating skills during the consultation. The investigators found that when patients were more controlling, expressed more emotion (of a negative kind), gave less information and were more effective in eliciting information from the doctor, at follow-up the diabetics had lower blood glucose (HbA1), and the hypertensives had lower diastolic blood pressure levels.

The method and results of this work are fascinating, as they question conventional approaches to change and previous assumptions about the relationship between process and outcome. It may at first seem counter-intuitive that the expression of negative emotion is associated with a better outcome. Most doctors will recall consultations in which issues were confronted in a way which were in the short run uncomfortable, but in the long run this seemed to lead to a better outcome for the patient. Perhaps some of Byrne and Long's (1976) 'dysfunctional' consultations in fact achieved better outcomes!

Evaluating the learning of communication skills

Do doctors learn from experience? More precisely, can they learn from experience without feedback? And, if they cannot, how can doctors improve their interviewing technique and demonstrate change in a quantifiable way? Byrne and Long (1976), Tuckett *et al.* (1985) and Verby *et al.* (1979) found that older doctors showed no consistent evidence of having better interviewing skills than younger doctors. From this evidence, it can be inferred that experience *per se* did not result in improved interviewing techniques. Byrne and Long found that doctors tended to use one style of interview technique, and this did not vary much from one consultation to the next. This occurred despite presumed variation in patients' needs. Tuckett *et al.* compared the performance of senior GP teachers and course organizers with other GPs. They found no measurable difference in the skill of the two groups as interviewers.

Walker (1988) evaluated a part-time trainers' course which took place over 1 year. The course organizers paid particular attention to changes in attitude, and to trainers becoming more patient-centred. No measurement of consultation skills was undertaken routinely as part of the course. As part of his research, Walker tested a sample of the trainers' consultations before and after the course, using Byrne and Long's 'doctor-centred, patient-centred' grid. He found that at the end of the course there was no significant shift in the doctors' behaviour, and they were, if anything, slightly more 'doctor-centred'! From this evidence, it might be inferred that it is not possible to assess the extent to which teachers' aims correspond to what learners learn and practise except by actually measuring the outcomes in question.

It may seem that teaching communication skills is rather like the blind leading the blind. Is there evidence that doctors can metaphorically pull themselves up by their bootlaces, and learn to be better interviewers? In Cardiff, Verby *et al.* (1979) set out to measure whether peer review by GPs of their videotaped consultations could improve their interviewing technique. A comparison group of GPs submitted videotapes, without meeting to discuss their tapes with colleagues. The investigators found that the peer learning group did improve their use of some behaviours measured on an independently developed assessment scale. The doctors picked up more leads, clarified more, used more facilitation, improved their questioning style and ended the interview more smoothly than the comparison group. The doctors who improved their consulting technique increased their consulting time significantly.

Measuring skill acquisition

Over a third of attenders in general practice may have an emotional problem. These problems are associated with longer consultations, missed diagnosis, frequent attendance and lack of agreement between doctor and patient about what the problem is. It is not surprising in this context that psychiatrists want to contribute to improving GPs' skills as interviewers. Gask *et al.* (1988) have applied a method which was initially developed at McMaster University in Canada by Lesser (1983). Interdisciplinary teaching there had allowed psychiatrists and general practitioners to develop a common training approach. Gask used a group of experienced GPs and gave them a course on communication using, as a substrate, their own videotaped interviews. After the course, the GPs applied some communication techniques with increased frequency. They used significantly more direct psychosocial questions and clarifying comments. The investigators also showed that a trainee group could change their behaviour using this method, and that the trainees who had below average skills at the outset improved the most.

Gask and her colleagues (1991) used their method to teach trainers, as this might have the greatest 'ripple effect' on future GPs. In order to measure the effect of learning about psychiatric interviewing skills on their teaching style, trainers provided videotapes of their tutorials with trainees before and after doing the course. Gask *et al.* found that after trainers had learned the new interviewing method, they provided more teaching during trainee tutorials on the picking up of verbal and non-verbal cues and making good eye contact. Trainers also employed more 'cue-based' teaching with their trainees. The intervention which produced the greatest impact on trainers' teaching behaviour was watching their own videotaped consultations in a group setting and being given feedback on their own consultation behaviour by the group.

From the combined evidence provided by Gask *et al.*'s studies, it can be inferred that GPs can improve their skills if they share and discuss their own taped consultations with a peer group and a facilitator. This is relatively labour-intensive and is therefore an expensive educational process. In the 1980s, the method of reimbursement of educational costs for doctors permitted interactive and relatively labour-intensive learning in groups. In the 1990s, reimbursement is no longer in proportion to the cost of the course, and it is not clear to what extent this type of learning will continue. This may be a practical barrier to further development. A second challenge is for GPs to develop and 'own' educational programmes designed to improve interviewing skills, which involve measurement and feedback as part of the training process.

References

Bain, D. J. G. (1976) Doctor–patient communications in general practice consultations. *Medical Education* 10: 125–131.

Balint, M. (1957) *The Doctor, his Patient and the Illness.* London: Tavistock.

Byrne, P. & Long, B. (1976) *Doctors Talking to Patients.* London: HMSO.

Francis, V., Korsch, B. M. & Morris, M. J. (1969) Gaps in doctor–patient communication. *New England Journal of Medicine* 280: 535–540.

Gask, L., Goldberg, D., Lesser, A. & Millar, T. (1988) Improving the psychiatric skills of the general practice trainee: An evaluation of a group training course. *Medical Education* 22: 132–138.

Gask, L., Goldberg, D., Boardman, J., Craig, T., Goddard, C., Jones, O., Kiseley, S., McGrath, G. & Millar, T. (1991) Training general practitioners to teach psychiatric interviewing skills: An evaluation of group training. *Medical Education* 25: 444–451.

Greenfield, S., Kaplan, S. H., Ware, J. E., Yano, E. M. & Frank, H. J. L. (1988) Patients' participation in medical care. *Journal of General Internal Medicine* 3: 448–457.

Henbest, R. J. & Stewart, M. (1990) Patient-centredness in the consultation: Does it really make a difference? *Family Practice* 7: 28–33.

Howie, J. G. R., Porter, A. M. D., Heaney, D. J. & Hopton, J. L. (1991) Long to short consultation ratio: A proxy measure of quality of care for general practice. *British Journal of General Practice* 41: 48–54.

Lesser, A. L. (1983) Problem-based interviews in general practice: A model. *Medical Education* 19: 299–304.

Maslow, A. H. (1970) *Motivation and Personality.* New York: Harper & Row.

Neighbour, R. (1987) *The Inner Consultation.* Lancaster: MTP Press Limited.

Pendleton, D., Schofield, T., Tate, P. & Havelock, P. (1984) *The Consultation: An Approach to Learning and Teaching.* Oxford: Oxford University Press.

Roter, D. L. (1977) Patient participation in patient–provider interaction: The effects of patient question-asking on the quality of interaction, satisfaction, and compliance. *Health Education Monographs* 5: 281–315.

Stewart, M. & Roter, D. (1989) (eds) *Communicating with Medical Patients.* Newbury Park: Sage Publications.

Stott, N. C. H. & Davis, R. H. (1979) The exceptional potential in each primary care consultation. *Journal of the Royal College of General Practitioners* 29: 201–205.

Tuckett, D., Boulton, M., Olson, C. & Williams, A. (1985) *Meetings Between Experts: An Approach to Sharing Ideas in Medical Consultations.* London: Tavistock Publications.

Verby, J. E., Holden, P. & Davis, R. H. (1979) Peer review of consultations in primary care: The use of audiovisual recordings. *British Medical Journal* 1: 1686–1688.

Walker, M. (1988) Training the trainers: Socialization and change in general practice. *Sociology of Health and Illness* 10: 282–302.

7

Screening for Carcinoma of the Cervix

> Mrs Dodds, aged 45, came to the surgery complaining of bleeding after intercourse. She had moved house often, and so had never had a cervical smear.

> Mrs Smart asked, 'What is mild dyskaryosis?' She had been asked to have a repeat smear in 6 months time and wondered if it was important whether she might go privately now.

Introduction

These two patients' problems illustrate the kind of problems and questions which doctors frequently get asked. In the first case, it seemed that a patient had not been offered or had not received any preventive service for cervical cancer until it was too late. The second patient had been made anxious about an abnormality found on screening. When doctors offer preventive services 'off their own bat' this raises important questions. Cochrane and Holland (1971) summarized the issues as follows.

> 'We believe there is an ethical difference between everyday medical practice and screening. If a patient asks a medical practitioner for help, the doctor does the best he can. He is not responsible for defects in medical knowledge. If, however, the practitioner initiates screening procedures, he is in a very different position. He should, in our view, have conclusive evidence that screening can alter the natural history of disease in a significant proportion of those screened.'

To screen or not to screen is therefore partially an ethical question, but the answer to the question depends on having a set of criteria against which the effectiveness of an intervention can be assessed. In order to do this in the case of cervical screening, the doctor needs to bring together knowledge from several disciplinary perspectives:

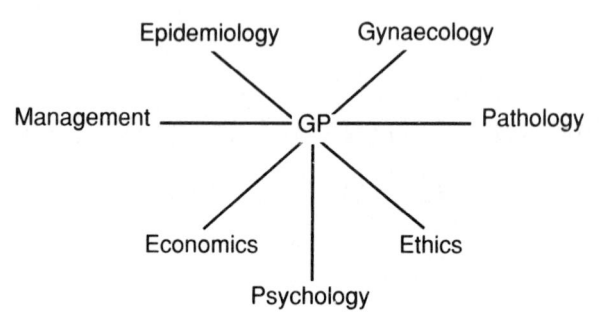

```
      Epidemiology      Gynaecology
               \       /
  Management ——— GP ——— Pathology
               /   |   \
         Economics |   Ethics
              Psychology
```

This chapter will address the following questions:
1. To what extent does cervical screening satisfy the criteria of effectiveness?
2. What are the barriers to effective screening?
3. What potential improvements can be made?

To what extent does cervical screening satisfy criteria of effectiveness?

Wilson and Jungner's screening criteria (1968) are a useful framework with which to assess the effectiveness of a screening method. Each criterion will be discussed with reference to cervical screening in order to critically assess its value in practice.

The disease

Is cervical carcinoma an important health problem?
The extent to which a disease poses a health problem can be measured in at least two ways. The mortality rate is one indicator. In 1984, 1899 women in England and Wales died of cervical carcinoma; 94 per cent of them were aged 35 and over (Office of Population Censuses and Surveys, 1985). This is the equivalent to three patients on the average GP's list dying of cervical carcinoma during his or her working life.

Death is the ultimate measure of ill-health, but some women will be diagnosed and cured, so not all women will die of their disease. In 1984, 4043 new cases of carcinoma of the cervix were diagnosed (OPCS, 1988). Approximately twice as many women are diagnosed with the disease as die of it in any one year. More women have lesions which are not invasive. In 1984, 8423 women were reported to have carcinoma *in situ* (OPCS, 1988), that is four times the number who were dying of invasive disease.

Table 7.1 *Statistics for cervical carcinoma 1984.*

Death from cervical carcinoma	1,899
Carcinoma of the cervix	4,043
Carcinoma *in situ*	8,423

Is the natural history of the disease well understood?
The natural history of cervical carcinoma is not well understood. Evidence derived by association suggests that cervical carcinoma is linked to an agent transmitted during sexual intercourse (Campion et al., 1986). The first changes occur at the transformation zone which lies between the squamous epithelium of the ectocervix and the columnar epithelium of the endocervix.

Cells which are superficial to the basement membrane in the transformation zone, illustrated below, may undergo neoplastic change. Histopathologists classify cervical intraepithelial neoplasia (CIN) on the basis of severity as CIN 1, 2 and 3. When neoplastic changes are found to extend deep to the epithelial basement membrane, invasive carcinoma is diagnosed.

CIN and carcinoma *in situ* are most frequently diagnosed in women aged 25–44; invasive carcinoma and deaths occur most frequently in women over 60 years of age, but it is difficult to infer the natural history of the disease because:

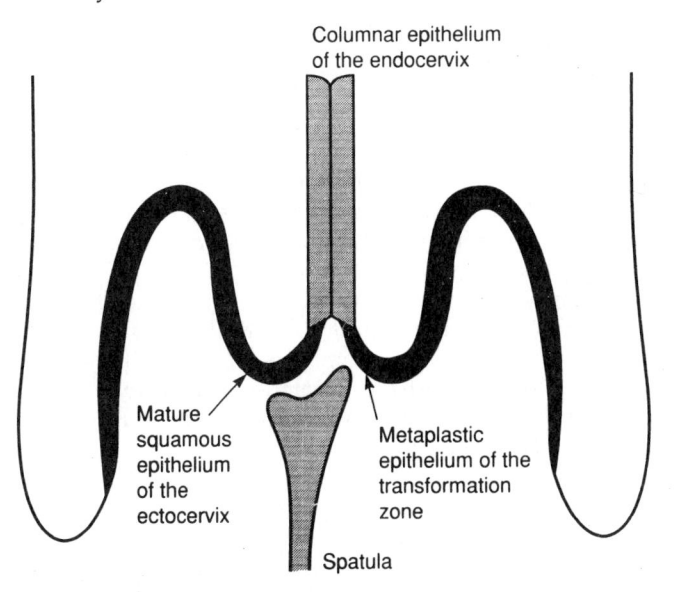

Fig. 7.1 Sampling the cervical transformation zone. (From Woodman et al., 1989. By permission of The Lancet Ltd.)

1. The identification of pre-clinical disease depends on the intensity of screening. It is likely that more CIN and carcinoma *in situ* will be identified in those who have been more extensively screened, for example young women.

2. The natural history of cervical cancer has been affected by pre-clinical identification and by medical management. Cook and Draper (1984) found that in some age groups there is evidence of a large increase in carcinoma *in situ*, but mortality had remained stable. They inferred that it is likely that a potential increase in cervical cancer incidence and mortality has been partially prevented as a result of the screening programme.

Is there a recognizable early stage?
The purpose of screening is to identify women before they reach the stage of clinically invasive carcinoma. Screening would ideally identify all women with carcinoma *in situ* or CIN3. The ideal diagnostic technique to identify CIN 3 would be colposcopy, with histological examination of clinically suspicious areas. This test is the gold standard. Screening involves the examination of a sample of exfoliated cervical cells. Cytologists make a prediction from this about the likely histological abnormality.

Table 7.2 *Identification of cervical intraepithelial neoplasia.*

Cytologist's report	Likely histology
Mild dysplasia predicts	CIN 1
Moderate dysplasia predicts	CIN 2
Severe dysplasia predicts	CIN 3 or carcinoma *in situ*

As cells beneath the basement membrane do not normally exfoliate, severe cytological dysplasia does not exclude the possibility of finding invasive carcinoma when a biopsy specimen is sent for histological examination (Evans *et al.*, 1986).

The finding of severe dysplasia is a recognizable early stage, identifiable through screening. It is likely that not all carcinoma *in situ* invades the basement membrane; a small proportion may regress. As clinicians believe that the risk of invasion is high, women with this condition are generally treated with laser therapy or other destructive therapy.

The screen

Is there a suitable test?
The initial diagnosis of cervical carcinoma is made by the histological examination of a biopsy specimen. Subsequent clinical staging depends on the degree of spread.

The screening test involves visualizing the cervix and collecting exfoliated cells by rotating a spatula twice over the surface. The sample is examined cytologically. Inevitably, there is loss of accuracy in using a simple test. The reasons for this are:

1. Small localized CIN lesions may fail to exfoliate sufficient abnormal cells (Giles et al., 1988).

2. The adequacy of samples is dependent on the presence of metaplastic and columnar cells of endocervical origin (Woodman et al., 1989). Gynaecologists, general practitioners and nurses vary in their ability to submit adequate smears (Duguid, 1986).

3. In older women the transformation zone moves into the os. In order to reach this area, a spatula with a pointed and extended tip (Wolfendale et al., 1987) or a spatula together with an endocervical brush (Taylor et al., 1987) should be used. When smears taken by many practitioners were compared, 22 per cent more smears with dyskaryotic cells were obtained with the spatula with a pointed and extended tip than with Ayre's spatula; and the cellular quality was significantly improved (Wolfendale, 1991). These instruments, illustrated below, are most effective in older women who are also at greater risk from cervical carcinoma.

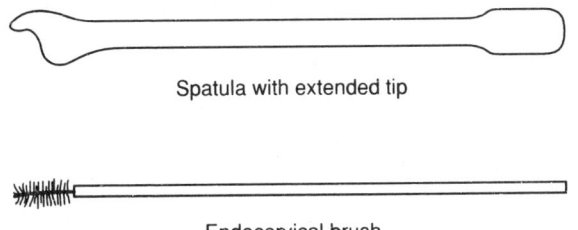

Spatula with extended tip

Endocervical brush

Fig. 7.2 Spatula with extended tip and endocervical brush. (From Wolfendale et al., 1987. By permission of *The British Medical Journal*.)

4. The recognition and grading of cell samples may vary from one cytologist to another and when cytologists are given the same samples to report on a second time. For these reasons, smear tests tend to underestimate the presence of disease (Chomet, 1987). A single smear has a false negative rate of about 40 per cent. However, after two independent tests, on average only 16 per cent of lesions will be negative on both occasions (IARC Working Group, 1986).

Is the test acceptable?
Some women do not accept the invitation to attend for cervical screening. The reasons for non-acceptance are practical, cognitive, attitudinal and emotional.

1. There is a higher uptake of screening if a specific appointment time is given (Wilson and Leeming, 1987). Some women find the time allocated inconvenient because of work or domestic commitments, or because they have a period on that date. The service requires built-in flexibility in order to allow women to telephone and change their appointment time.

2. Some women do not know or understand the reasons for cervical screening. McAvoy and Raza (1991) found that Asian women lacked knowledge and had a particularly low uptake of cervical screening. Personal visits to provide health education, particularly with videotaped information, increased the uptake of screening by this group significantly. Where there is medical uncertainty about the benefits of a procedure, patients will also be uncertain. Some patients think they are ineligible, because they associate the disease with promiscuity, when they themselves have had only one sexual partner (Meadows, 1987) or believe they need a current sexual partner to be at risk. They may not realize that there is a need for continued monitoring, or they may be confused about the varying intervals recommended.

3. A third reason for refusal is attitudinal. Some people dislike medical intervention of any kind. Some have a fatalistic attitude or fear the discovery of cancer (Nathoo, 1988).

4. Embarrassment about an internal examination deters some women. When they have never had a smear, most of them express a preference for the procedure to be done by female personnel (Standing and Mercer, 1984). This preference is more strongly held by ethnic groups such as Asians (McAvoy and Raza, 1988). This kind of response has been recorded by interviewing non-responders:

> 'No, I did not go – I just keep putting it off and putting it off. It is embarrassing. You see the last time I had it done – my doctor is a man doctor, and I just don't feel it is right that a man should be doing that kind of thing – I don't think men should do it ... it is just too embarrassing' (Elkind et al., 1988).

Reasons for non-acceptance, when known by the providers, can be circumvented. Non-acceptance is sometimes assumed to be a major obstacle to cervical screening. However, provided that patients' practical, cognitive and emotional needs are met, only about 10 per cent of women will refuse (Standing and Mercer, 1984; Ridsdale, 1987).

At what intervals should screening be repeated?
The purpose of screening is to identify abnormalities before they become clinically apparent. The duration of the detectable pre-clinical phase is known as the sojourn time. Ideally, monitoring would

occur at sufficiently frequent intervals to detect abnormal cytology during this sojourn time.

Data from European and North American studies have been pooled to assess the optimal frequency of screening. It has been estimated from these data that if all women had at least one screen prior to the age of 35, and were then re-screened at 5-year intervals, there would be an 84 per cent reduction in the cumulative incidence of invasive cervical cancer. Screening at 3-year intervals would reduce the cumulative incidence by 91 per cent (IARC Working Group, 1986).

A more difficult question is: at what intervals should women be rescreened when the cytologists report moderate dyskaryosis? Fox (1987) argued that if colposcopy services were freely available, then all women with these abnormalities would benefit from the service. As cytological predictions tend to underestimate abnormalities found on colposcopy, if moderate dyskaryosis is reported, the patient should be referred for colposcopy.

The natural history and management of mild dyskaryosis are controversial. Follow-up of these women shows that up to 26 per cent will progress to CIN 3 in 2 years (Campion *et al.*, 1986). But in the same period up to half can revert to normal (Robertson *et al.*, 1988). In view of the high frequency of this abnormality, the variable outcome and scarce resources, recommendations vary from colposcopy to a repeat smear in 6 months or 1 year.

Follow-up

Are there adequate facilities for the diagnosis and treatment of detected abnormalities?

Bottle-necks in the provision of services can occur from the GP's surgery, when patients find telephone lines engaged, through to waiting lists for colposcopy clinics and for admission to hospital. The extent to which facilities are judged adequate also depends on clinical opinion about the appropriate stage at which cytological abnormalities require further investigation. There is agreement that severe dysplasia on cytology requires referral for diagnosis and treatment.

The management of patients whose smear is reported as mild or moderately dysplastic is more controversial. If cytologists recommended that GPs refer all women for cytology when moderate dysplasia is first reported, there would be bottle-necks in the system. Cytologists therefore base their recommendations on pragmatic considerations locally. Patients with moderate dysplasia may be asked to return for a repeat smear in a prescribed period or they may be referred for colposcopy straight away (BSCC Working Party, 1986).

Reducing pressure on colposcopy clinics increases pressure on the provision and organization of cytology services. In order to link information obtained on sequential smears and inform doctors and patients of the results, laboratories need computer systems. If results are not linked, a patient with a normal smear may be asked to return in 3 years when a smear done previously showed moderate dyskaryosis.

If all women in the United Kingdom with mild dyskaryosis were referred for colposcopy, the present NHS facilities for diagnosis and treatment would not be adequate.

Is treatment of the disease at an early stage of more benefit than treatment started at a later stage?

One outcome measure of benefit is avoided mortality. A randomized controlled study of cervical screening has not been undertaken, but some populations have been offered systematic cervical screening over the past few decades, whilst others have not. Provided that risk factors for cervical cancer do not act differentially between countries, then changes in mortality will indicate the benefit of early identification and treatment.

In Iceland there is a nationwide programme with a wide target age range. Between 1965 and 1982 mortality fell by 80 per cent (Laara *et al.*, 1987). Finland has a smaller target age range and less frequent screening intervals. There was a 50 per cent reduction in mortality over the same period. In Norway, with only 5 per cent of the population covered by organized screening, mortality fell by only 10 per cent. During the same period, the decline in mortality from cervical cancer in Britain was 21 per cent. This evidence supports the concept that the presence and extent of screening is associated with a decrease in mortality from cervical carcinoma.

Screening for carcinoma *in situ* could also prevent morbidity from clinically invasive disease. A systematic screening programme to detect pre-invasive carcinoma of the cervix was started in British Columbia in 1949. Between 1955 and 1985, the incidence of invasive squamous carcinoma of the cervix fell by 78 per cent (Anderson *et al.*, 1988). This was during a time in which there was an appreciable increase in carcinoma *in situ*. This evidence suggests that morbidity can also be prevented.

A third way to assess the potential benefit of screening (or loss to women not identified) is examination of the screening status of women who have developed cancer. La Vecchia and colleagues (1984) found that women who had undergone two or more smears were more likely to have had their cancer diagnosed at an early stage, and lack of screening was associated with more advanced stage cancers. In a study of women who died, 90 per cent had never been screened (Spriggs and Boddington, 1976).

A final way to test whether treatment at an early stage would be more beneficial is not to treat patients with abnormalities, but to continue monitoring them. This was done by Green in New Zealand (Flagler and Winkler, 1992). The design and ethics of this study were the subject of a judicial review. Flagler and Winkler discussed the issues raised and reported that progression to subsequent invasive cancer occurred in 29 out of 131 (22 per cent) women with abnormal smears, and in 12 out of 817 (1.5 per cent) women with normal smears. The progression rate to cervical cancer for those patients with persistent abnormal cytology was ten times higher than it was for those with negative follow-up cytology.

Ethics

Are the chances of physical and psychological harm less than the chance of benefit?
The doctor has both a duty to do no harm (non-maleficence), and a duty which involves the prevention and removal of harm (beneficence). Two other basic principles are respect for autonomy and the principle of justice (Beauchamp and Childress, 1983). The principles of medical ethics will be discussed more fully in Chapter 8.

Illich (1976) argued that western societies are undermining personal autonomy by medicalizing life. Skrabenek (1988) argued that screening for cervical cancer, in particular, is an act of unwarranted medicalization. Whether it is warranted depends to a certain extent on an estimate of the benefit which has been, or may be, achieved. If the Icelandic and British Columbian results were reproduced in Britain, approximately 1,600 out of 2,000 lives might be saved, and 3,200 out of 4,000 invasive cancers might be prevented each year.

Against benefits and potential benefits, physical and psychological harms need to be weighed. Patients with mild and moderate dysplasia are made anxious (Reelick *et al.*, 1984), and treatment may cause physical and psychological harm (Britten, 1988; Posner and Vessey, 1988). Unsystematic screening may incur harm without sufficient benefit. The reductions in mortality and morbidity were achieved in Iceland and British Columbia with systematic screening. If this outcome is possible with systematic screening in the UK, then it would seem fair to inform every woman in the population and offer her screening. The benefit rate in terms of preventing disease and mortality is more likely to increase when all women are systematically informed and invited.

Economics

Can the cost be balanced against the benefits the service provides, and against other opportunity costs and benefits?
There have been very few attempts to measure the costs and

benefits of cervical screening. In the mid-1980s, the Department of Health estimated the cost of undertaking and reporting a smear to be between £5 and £15.40. Assuming an average cost of £10, 4.5 million smears would cost £45 million. In 1984, 94 per cent of deaths and 45 per cent of the screening occurred in the over 35s; 6 per cent of deaths and 55 per cent of the screening occurred in the under 35s. Translating this into figures of investment for avoidable mortality, approximately £20 million was spent in an attempt to prevent 1,785 deaths in the over 35s, whilst £25 million was spent attempting to avoid 114 deaths in the under 35s. In other words, approximately £10,000 was being spent per avoidable death on older women, but £220,000 was being spent per avoidable death on the under 35s.

Because of the high cost to benefit ratio, some economists (Roberts et al., 1985) have pointed out that the same investment would prevent more deaths in other areas of the NHS. However, the high cost per life saved in the 1980s reflected the fact that the group with the lower risk were screened most intensively and frequently. High cost and low effectiveness are not an inevitable outcome of cervical screening. They are the consequence of an unplanned and poorly distributed service. Using a computer simulation model, Parkin and Moss (1986) suggested that 5-yearly testing of women aged over 35 is the most cost-effective option. Van Oortmarssen et al. (1992) estimated from Dutch data that 5-yearly screening for women aged 37–62 would have a cost-effectiveness ratio of £8,000 per life year saved, assuming a comparatively low uptake of 65 per cent. Extension of screening to women in lower risk groups or an increase in the frequency of screening leads to a progressive reduction in the marginal benefit per unit cost.

What are the barriers to effective screening?

Wilson and Jungner's (1968) criteria have been used to examine the performance of cervical screening. There is a lack of scientific knowledge about the epidemiology and pathology of cervical carcinoma, which makes clinical decision-making difficult. However, the complexity of this area need not lead to reductive or nihilistic thinking, but to clinicians continuing to evaluate new evidence with an open mind. One challenge is to identify obstacles to a systematic service and find solutions for them. One hundred cases of invasive cervical cancer were reviewed by Ellman and Chamberlain (1984) in order to assess how screening might be improved. The results are illustrated in Figure 7.3. They found:

1. In 68 cases, no screening had been undertaken.
2. In 13 cases, suspicious cervical smear reports had not been followed up adequately.

Screening for carcinoma of the cervix

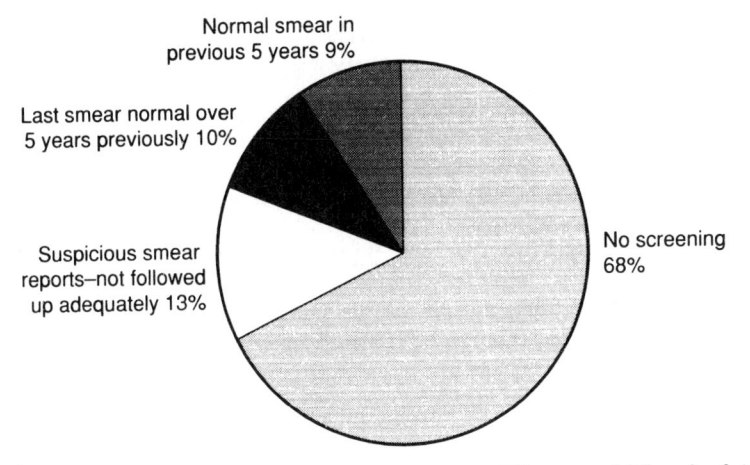

Fig. 7.3 Review of 100 cervical cancer cases. (Fom Ellman and Chamberlain, 1984.)

3. In ten cases, the last smear was reported as normal over 5 years previously.
4. In nine cases, a normal smear had been reported in the last 5 years.

The care of these groups will be considered in turn:

1. Sixty-eight per cent of women with invasive cancer had never received screening. How can this be explained? In the 1980s there were no national figures for screening rates, but regional surveys (Charney and Lewis, 1987; Coulter and Baldwin, 1987) showed approximately 50–75 per cent of women reported having had a smear in the previous 5 years. Women with invasive carcinoma, however, were more likely to be older, widowed or divorced (Sansom et al., 1971) and living in more deprived areas (Johnson et al., 1987). Women whose age, civil status and class put them at greater risk were less likely to have been screened. A survey in one region illustrates the two ends of the range. Ninety per cent of women in social class 1 and 2 aged 25–34 were reported as having had smears in the previous 5 years, whilst 44 per cent of women in social class 4 and 5 aged 55–64 had undergone a smear in the previous 5 years (Coulter and Baldwin, 1987).

Charny and Lewis (1987) asked a group of women why they had never been screened. The most frequent response was that they had not been asked. A useful model of utilization of screening services, illustrated in Figure 7.4, has been developed by Eardley et al. (1985).

Self-initiators are likely to be middle class and knowledgeable about the potential of screening to prevent cancer. In the context of the failure of spontaneous screening to reach a large proportion of

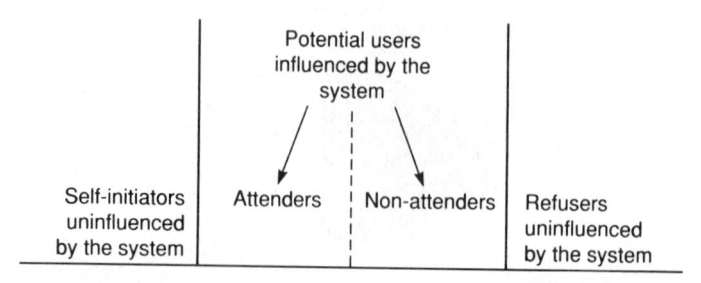

```
|Self-initiators    | Potential users         | Refusers        |
|uninfluenced       | influenced by the       | uninfluenced    |
|by the system      | system                  | by the system   |
|                   |  ↙        ↘             |                 |
|                   | Attenders | Non-attenders |               |
```

Fig. 7.4 Model of utilization of cervical screening. (From Eardley *et al.*, 1985. With kind permission from Elsevier Science Ltd.)

women at risk, the decision to adopt a universal programme to invite women was an advance, but operating this system has identified other barriers. In urban areas it has been found that up to one-half of patients are no longer at the address they gave when registering (Beardow *et al.*, 1989). In addition, when invitations are sent without women having sufficient information about their eligibility and the purpose of the test, the response rate may be low.

Standing and Mercer (1984) found 60 per cent of women preferred to see a female health professional for cervical screening, but in 1987 over 10,000 GPs serving over 20 million patients had no woman partner (Department of Health, 1989). Some practices may have had a salaried woman doctor or nurse available, but those who did not would have been less likely to have women agreeing to be screened, particularly in the case of those who had never had a cervical smear or those who belonged to some religious or ethnic subgroups.

2. In Ellman and Chamberlain's (1985) study, 13 per cent of women with invasive carcinoma had had suspicious smears reported which had not been adequately followed up. The most frequent reason for poor follow-up was that the patient moved to a new and unknown address. Lack of computer systems which can link patients' results with previous smears and improve communication between the laboratory and GPs was another cause of failure of follow-up.

3. Ten per cent of women with invasive carcinoma had had normal smears performed more than 5 years previously. It is likely that these women did not know they required repeat monitoring, and that they had not been recalled by the system then in operation. In an analysis of the national recall system Pye (1988) estimated that only 3 per cent of the appropriate population were effectively recalled by the recall system.

4. Nine per cent of patients had had normal smear reports within 5 years of their diagnosis of invasive cancer. It was estimated that half of these might have been due to false negative reports.

What potential improvements can be made?

1. The introduction of a universal call and recall scheme based on FHSA computer systems was a step forward. There was already evidence from a single practice experiment that systematic invitations increased the use of the service by those who had not previously been screened (Pierce et al., 1989). Reid et al. (1991) in Scotland found that after a call programme was begun 26 practices improved their mean screening level for women aged 20–60 from 71 per cent to 78 per cent. Six months after the new contract with its incentives to achieve targets, the level of those screened was further improved to a mean of 85 per cent. The practice lists were inflated by an average 4 per cent, so the mean true population coverage was almost 90 per cent.

2. It has been shown that patients are more likely to respond if offered specific appointment times. FHSAs therefore need to improve communications with local practices, and practices need to provide flexibility for those wishing to change their appointments.

3. Women who are invited should receive information, as shown in Figure 7.5, in booklets about the purpose of the test and its applicability to the recipient (Eardley et al., 1988). Wilkinson et al. (1990) have shown that when abnormalities were found on screening, a personal letter and an explanatory leaflet produced less anxiety in women being recalled than a standard computerized letter.

4. In view of patients' expressed preference that screening be undertaken by women doctors or nurses, every practice needs to ensure that appropriate personnel are available. Before the 1990 contract, some doctors were unwilling to delegate smear testing to trained nurses. One rationale was that doctors may screen for ovarian pathology by simultaneously performing a bimanual examination. However, Williams (1992) found that no studies of early detection of ovarian carcinoma had demonstrated improved survival rates, even when ultrasound or Doppler techniques were used, and there seems little point in identifying benign asymptomatic lesions.

5. There is some evidence that after the new economic incentives provided by the 1990 contract, some nurses were delegated this and other tasks without training (Ross et al., 1994). All practitioners require initial training, and they also need feedback from the laboratory on the quality of the samples they obtain in relation to their peers. If performance is improved, this will decrease the rate of false negative reports.

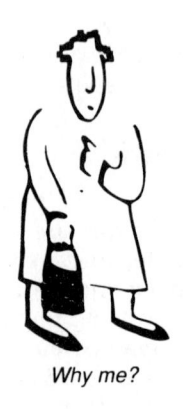

Why invite me?
All women between the ages of 20 and 64 are now being invited every 5 years

Isn't it just for young women?
No, in fact it is most important that women over 35 who have never had the test before should have one done

What if I'm past the change of life?
Even after the menopause women need to be tested regularly to make sure that the cervix is still healthy

Why me?

Why should I have the test? There's nothing wrong with me
The idea of the test is to find small changes that might cause problems later on, so that they can be dealt with before you get any symptoms

What if I've had a hysterectomy?
Some women who have had a hysterectomy still need to have a test. So ask your doctor what is right for you

What if I've had the test in the last five years?
If you think you are not due for another test check with your doctor or at the clinic

So are there any women who don't need a test?
All women would really benefit from having the test – even women who sometimes think they don't need the test any more such as widows and divorced women

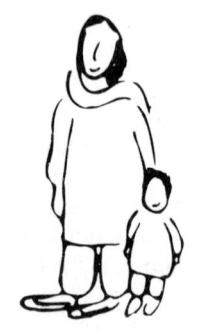

Do I need a test?

Fig. 7.5 Extract from the new edition of *You're invited* (From Eardley *et al.*, 1988. By permission of the Health Education Authority.)

6. Cytology laboratories need computer systems to process information, and continuing quality assessment in order to minimize false negatives.

7. Family Health Service Authorities (FHSAs) must agree nationally on the frequency with which women require surveillance, as different policies cause confusion for patients and their doctors.

8. Operating the call scheme revealed the inadequacy of popula-

tion registers. If FHSA registers are inaccurate and this inaccuracy leads to a poor response to screening, more radical solutions may be considered. In some Swedish counties, each person is required to register a change of address with the parish in which they reside. This requirement is so interlocked with other government functions, including workers' compensation and health care, that compliance is virtually universal. With these registers, more than 90 per cent of the eligible population have attended for cervical screening (Stenkvist et al., 1984). To some, compulsory registration of change of address may seem to be excessively paternalistic. Others may see it as a necessary prerequisite if screening is to be cost-effective. These issues need to be discussed if screeners wish to create the political will to enable systems like those working in Sweden to be introduced in the UK.

Conclusion

Having considered the contributions of different disciplines to an understanding of cervical screening, the clinician returns to the patients.

1. Mrs Dodds, with post-coital bleeding, had never received an invitation for screening, as she had moved house within the practice. On examination there was a hard lump on her cervix. She had invasive carcinoma.

2. Mrs Smart-Jones had mild dyskaryosis. Rather than wait for a repeat smear in 6 months, she went to see a gynaecologist privately. She underwent colposcopy and laser treatment for CIN 2 and had a secondary haemorrhage.

References

Anderson, G. H., Boyes, D. A., Benedet, J. L. et al. (1988) Organization and results of the cervical cytology screening programme in British Columbia, 1955–85. *British Medical Journal* 296: 975–978.

Beardow, R., Oerton, J. & Victor, C. (1989) Evaluation of the cervical cytology screening programme in an inner city health district. *British Medical Journal* 299: 98–100.

Beauchamp, T. L. & Childress, J. F. (1983) *Principles of Biomedical Ethics*, 2nd edn. New York: Oxford University Press.

Britten, N. (1988) Personal view. *British Medical Journal* 296: 1191.

BSCC Working Party on Terminology in Gynaecological Cytopathology (1986) Management of women with abnormal cervical smears. *The Bulletin of the Royal College of Pathologists* 56: 1–2.

Campion, M. J., Cuzick, J., McCance, D. J. & Singer, A. (1986) Progressive potential of mild cervical atypia: Prospective cytological, colposcopic and virological study. *The Lancet ii*: 237–240.

Charney, M. C. & Lewis, P. A. (1987) Who is using cervical cancer screening services? *Health Trends* 19: 3–5.

Chomet, J. (1987) Screening for cervical cancer: A new scope for general practitioners? Results of the first year of colposcopy in general practice. *British Medical Journal* 294: 1326–1328.

Cochrane, A. L. & Holland, W. W. (1971) Validation of screening procedures. *British Medical Bulletin* 27: 3–8.

Cook, G. A. & Draper, G. J. (1984) Trends in cervical cancer and carcinoma in situ in Great Britain. *British Journal of Cancer* 50: 367–374.

Coulter, A. & Baldwin, A. (1987) Surveys of population coverage in cervical cancer screening in the Oxford region. *Journal of the Royal College of General Practitioners* 37: 441–443.

Department of Health (1989) Personal Communication.

Duguid, H. L. D. (1986) Does mild atypia on a cervical smear warrant further investigation? *The Lancet ii*: 1225.

Eardley, A., Elkind, A. K., Spencer, B., Hobbs, P., Pendleton, L. L. & Haran, D. (1985) Attendance for cervical screening – whose problem? *Social Science and Medicine* 20: 955–962.

Eardley, A., Alkind, A., Spencer, B., Haran, D., Hobbs, P. & McGuiness, H. (1988) Health Education in a computer-managed cervical screening programme. *Health Education Journal* 47: 43–47.

Elkind, A. K., Haran, D., Eardley, A. & Spencer, B. (1988) Reasons for non-attendance for computer-managed cervical screening: Pilot interviews. *Social Science and Medicine* 27: 651–660.

Ellman, R. & Chamberlain, J. (1984) Improving the effectiveness of cervical cancer screening. *Journal of the Royal College of General Practitioners* 34: 537–542.

Evans, D. J. D., Hudson, E. A., Brown, C. L. et al. (1986) Terminology in gynaecological cytopathology: Report of the working party of the British Society for Clinical Cytology. *Journal of Clinical Pathology* 39: 933–944.

Flagler, E. & Winkler, E. R. (1992) 'An unfortunate experiment': the New Zealand study of cancer of the cervix. *Annals of the Royal College of Physicians and Surgeons, Canada* 25: 124–130.

Fox, H. (1987) Cervical smears: New terminology and new demands. *British Medical Journal* 294: 1307–1308.

Giles, J. A., Hudson, E., Crow, J., Williams, D. & Walker, P. (1988) Colposcopic assessment of the accuracy of cervical cytology screening. *British Medical Journal* 296: 1099–1102.

IARC Working Group on evaluation of cervical cancer screening programmes (1986) Screening for squamous cervical cancer: Duration of low risk after negative results of cervical cytology and its implications for screening programmes. *British Medical Journal* 293: 656–664.

Illich, I. (1976) *Limits to Medicine. Medical Nemesis: The Expropriation of Health.* London: Boyars.

Johnson, I. S., Milner, P. C. & Todd, J. N. (1987) An assessment of the effectiveness of cervical cytology screening in Sheffield. *Community Medicine* 9: 160–170.

Laara, E., Day, N. E. & Hakama, M. (1987) Trends in mortality from cervi-

cal cancer in the Nordic countries: Association with organized screening programmes. *The Lancet i:* 1247–1249.
La Vecchia, C., Decavli, A., Gentile, A., Franceschi, S., Fasoli, M. & Tognoni, G. (1984) 'Pap' smear and the risk of cervical neoplasia: Quantitative estimates from a case–control study. *The Lancet ii:* 779–782.
McAvoy, B. R. & Raza, R. (1988) Contraceptive service and cervical cytology. *Health Trends* 20: 14–17.
McAvoy, B. R. & Raza, R. (1991) Can health education increase uptake of cervical smear testing among Asian women? *British Medical Journal* 302: 833–835.
Meadows, P. (1987) Study of the women overdue for a smear test in a general practice cervical screening programme. *Journal of the Royal College of General Practitioners* 37: 500–503.
Nathoo, V. (1988) Investigation of non-responders at a cervical cancer screening clinic in Manchester. *British Medical Journal* 296: 1041–1042.
Oortmarssen, G. J. van, Habbema, J., Dik, F. & Ballegooijen, M. van (1992). Predicting mortality from cervical cancer after negative smear test results. *British Medical Journal* 305: 449–451.
Office of Population Censuses and Surveys (OPCS) (1985) *Mortality Statistics by Cause: England and Wales 1984.* London: HMSO.
OPCS (1988) *Cancer Statistics Registrations: England and Wales 1984.* London: HMSO.
Parkin, D. M. & Moss, S. M. (1986) An evaluation of screening policies for cervical cancer in England and Wales using a computer simulation model. *Journal of Epidemiology and Community Health* 40: 143–153.
Pierce, M., Lundy, S., Palanisamy, A., Winning, S. & King, J. (1989) Prospective randomized controlled trial of methods of call and recall for cervical cytology screening. *British Medical Journal* 298: 160–162.
Posner, T. & Vessey, M. (1988) *Prevention of Cervical Cancer: The Patient's View.* London: King's Fund Publishing Office.
Pye, M. J. (1988) Screening for cervical cancer: Review of administrative arrangements. *Journal of the Royal Society of Medicine* 81: 82–83.
Reelick, N. F., de Haes, W. F. M. & Shuurman, J. H. (1984) Psychological side-effects of the mass screening on cervical cancer. *Social Science and Medicine* 18: 1089–1093.
Reid, G. S., Robertson, A. J., Bissett, C., Smith, J., Waugh, N. & Halkerston, R. (1991). Cervical screening in Perth and Kinross since introduction of the new contract. *British Medical Journal* 303: 447–450.
Ridsdale, L. L. (1987) Cervical screening in general practice: Call and recall. *Journal of the Royal College of General Practitioners* 37: 257–259.
Roberts, C. J., Charney, M. C. & Farrow, S. C. (1985) How much can the NHS afford to spend to save a life or avoid a severe disability? *The Lancet i:* 89–91.
Robertson, J. H., Woodend, B. E., Crozier, E. H. & Hutchinson, J. (1988) Risk of cervical cancer associated with mild dyskaryosis. *British Medical Journal* 297: 18–21.
Ross, F. M., Bower, P. J. & Sibbald, B. S. (1994) Practice nurses: characteristics, workload and training needs. *British Journal of General Practice* 44: 15–18.
Sansom, C. D., Wakefield, J. & Yule, R. (1971) Trends in cytological screening in the Manchester area 1965–71. *Community Medicine* 126: 253–257.

Skrabenek, P. (1988) The physician's responsibility to the patient. *The Lancet i:* 1155–1156.

Spriggs, A. I. & Boddington, M. M. (1976) Protection by cervical smears. *The Lancet i:* 143.

Standing, P. & Mercer, S. (1984) Quinquennial cervical smears: Every woman's right and every practitioner's responsibility. *British Medical Journal 289:* 883–886.

Stenkvist, B., Bergstrom, R., Eklund, G. & Fox, C. (1984) Papanicolaou smear screening and cervical cancer: What can you expect? *Journal of the American Medical Association 252:* 1423–1426.

Taylor, P. T., Andersen, W. A., Barber, S. R., Covell, B. L., Smith, E. B. & Underwood, P. B. (1987) The screening Papanicolaou smear: Contribution of the endocervical brush. *Obstetrics and Gynaecology 70:* 734–737.

Wilkinson, C., Jones, J. M. & McBride, J. (1990) Anxiety caused by abnormal result of cervical smear test: A controlled trial. *British Medical Journal 300:* 440.

Williams, C. (1992) Ovarian and cervical cancer. *British Medical Journal 304:* 1501–4.

Wilson, A. & Leeming, A. (1987) Cervical cytology screening: A comparison of two call systems. *British Medical Journal 295:* 181–182.

Wilson, J. M. G. & Jungner, G. (1968) *Principles and Practice of Screening for Disease.* WHO Public Health Paper no. 34. Geneva: World Health Organization.

Wolfendale, M. (1991) Cervical samplers: Most important variable is probably the operator's skill. *British Medical Journal 302:* 1554–5.

Wolfendale, M., Howe-Guest, R., Usherwood, M. & Draper, G. (1987) Controlled trial of a new cervical spatula. *British Medical Journal 294:* 33–35.

Woodman, C. B. J., Yates, M., Ward, K., Williams, D., Tomlinson, K. & Luesley, D. (1989) Indicators of effective cytological sampling of the uterine cervix. *The Lancet ii:* 88–90.

8

Medical Ethics

> Mrs Black came to see me about her 77-year-old mother-in-law, a patient of mine. She explained that she and her husband were worried about my patient's ability to drive. My patient evidently did not turn on her car lights at night and sometimes could not find the pedals. She never used indicators and claimed that she did not need to as *she* knew what she was going to do.

> Then a 44-year-old woman came to see me with a prescription for fertility drugs from a private doctor. She asked me to copy this onto an NHS prescription pad so that she could get the drugs at less expense.

Introduction

This chapter is concerned with how doctors reason when they are presented with conflicts of interest. Looking back on their medical training and experience in practice, almost every doctor will recognize times when they were asked to make judgements and decisions in situations which were conflictual. The conflicts may have occurred between patients and their relatives or friends, between patients and doctors or other medical professionals, or between different providers of health care. When situations like this occur, those responsible for participating in decision-making tend to feel stressed. Such conflicts require at least three components if they are to be resolved; <u>time</u>, <u>communication skills</u> and <u>knowledge of medical ethics</u>. The first two have been described in previous chapters. This chapter will focus on the rationale for decision-making in particular instances, and provide some tools and a framework for reasoning about issues involving medical ethics.

Medical ethics has not, until recently, been explicitly taught during medical training. And as long as training in the 'science' of medicine is separate from other faculties in British universities, it remains difficult for doctors to learn about the language and concepts which form the building blocks of subjects as taught in humanities and the social sciences. Discussion of ethics requires a framework and a language in the same way that medicine does. This language evolved as part of moral philosophy. Two major ways of approaching moral judgements are advocated in philosophy. In practice, the difference between the two is not great.

Utilitarianism

One school of philosophers, the utilitarians, look at the outcomes or consequences of actions in a way which is similar to that of epidemiologists. Decisions made according to this way of thinking need to be justified by their ability to maximize good outcomes for everybody. This utilitarian approach has been simplified into maxims like 'promoting the greatest good of the greatest number' and the somewhat pejoratively used epithet 'the end justifies the means' (Beauchamp and Childress, 1983).

Deontology

The second approach has a rather cumbersome name, deontology. Like many medical words, it derives from a Greek term *deon*, meaning duty. The duties or principles which should guide reasoning are the subject of debate. Doctors have traditionally accepted two duties. One is of not inflicting harm (non-maleficence), and the second is to benefit patients (beneficence). These principles are closely related to the estimated consequences of actions which are prioritized in utilitarianism.

Russell (1984) and Scruton (1982) have described the evolution of a third principle, *autonomy*. Like other philosophical (and medical) words, it is derived from Greek meaning self-rule. But the concept developed a major place in philosophy through the work of Kant. Kant derived a theory of duty applicable to all persons which is similar to the religious maxim 'do as you would be done by'. His idea was that people should act as if whatever they did would become a general law. This conceptual process of putting oneself on the receiving end, as well as in the active role, is useful; even a burglar would be angry to find that his house had been burgled. A component of this principle is that each person must be treated as an end, and never as a means to other ends. The application of this principle may run counter to utilitarianism. The medical profession has traditionally tended to be paternalistic, but respecting patients' autonomy is now given more prominence and priority in the debate about medical ethics.

A fourth principle which is also sometimes difficult for doctors to come to terms with is one of *justice* or fairness towards all people when allocating resources, including medical care. Rawls (1971) argued that a fair contract could be made between people on the allocation of resources if the contractors had no advance knowledge of their talents and abilities, and presumably also their future illnesses and handicaps.

These four principles are the foundation stones of medical ethics. How they should be applied in complex medical situations, and which should be given priority when there is conflict, is the subject of debate.

Doctors and drivers

The first case presented above is one in which the family had asked me, the doctor, to 'blow the whistle' on an elderly patient and effectively end her career as an independent driver. My first reaction was to look at the patient's notes. She had had few medical problems in the past, but 2 years ago I had noted that she was forgetful, confused, mild to moderately demented, still driving and not wanting to move out of her home before she died. After listening to the daughter-in-law's comments, I asked Mrs Black to come and see me again, confirmed my previous impression that she was mildly to moderately demented, and arranged for tests to rule out any treatable medical condition. During this and subsequent appointments, we discussed her driving and she said that she could manage on foot and by using public transport. But she did not seem to appreciate that her driving might cause increased risks to others and was reluctant voluntarily to relinquish her driving licence.

Every GP will have encountered a similar experience, and it places them in a double-bind. The licensing laws do not require repeat examinations either by doctors or by assessment of performance under test conditions. The law in Britain requires patients to self-declare conditions that might impair their ability to drive. However, for the patient, dementia is frequently accompanied either by loss of memory and cognitive ability, with a lack of ability to recognize the problem, or by denial and sometimes by inappropriate euphoria. People naturally cling to their right to drive, as this helps them to remain in their own homes and have self-initiated access to shops, friends and so on. As immobile patients lead to more work through home visiting, GPs are often tempted to collude with patients if they say they will only use the car to drive short distances during the day to visit the shops and the doctor. And doctors naturally want to maintain a relationship of trust with patients, which depends on keeping secret or in confidence the information they have about patients.

These issues will now be examined within the framework provided by medical ethics. When doctors and other decision-makers reason about the decisions they have to make, they can defend or justify decision-making in many ways. As the consequence of any decision or action is unforeseen at the time the judgement is made and cannot be predicted with certainty, one approach is to apply general principles irrespective of the consequences. The first, and arguably the most important, of these principles is to respect each person's freedom or autonomy to weigh up the risks and benefits of their own decisions and actions. And in order for them to be able to do this, the doctor's role is to inform patients as fully as possible of the scientific evidence. In this case, by continuing to drive, the patient presumably believed that she would derive the most benefit in terms of retaining her independence to live in her own home, do her own shopping and visit her friends at will. At some level she must have appreciated that she was incurring risks both to herself and others, but presumably she believed that the risks she was taking, at least the risk of harming herself, had a lower priority that the benefit she derived from continuing to drive.

From my point of view, the ideal outcome might have been that, having been informed of the risks of continuing to drive and the concerns expressed about her by others, the patient freely decided to volunteer for reassessment and, if necessary, give up driving. Some patients do agree to do this and others agree when they understand, as in the case of those with epilepsy, that their insurance will be invalidated by a failure to declare their condition. Nevertheless, it is reported that up to a fifth of patients with epilepsy continue to drive (Scambler, 1989). The guidelines are not absolutely clear on the subject of doctors' responsibility towards the general public with regard to patients who are becoming demented (Medical Advisory Branch DVLA, 1993).

Reasoning in this case would be influenced by clinical as well as by moral criteria. The clinical judgement would depend on one's ability to assess the patient's general knowledge and reasoning, and her ability to appraise and act on the information about her specific condition. It appeared to me that my patient's knowledge and reasoning seemed insufficient for her to judge the likely risks and consequences of her actions. If her actions only led to risks to herself, there would be less reason for not respecting her autonomy (Mill in Gillon, 1986). However, in this case her failure to disclose necessary information exposed others to the risk of death or serious harm.

Deciding about preventing harm to others is a difficult role for doctors to adopt, as clinicians generally think primarily of the person sitting in front of them. Moreover, risk of harm or death is extremely difficult to estimate. Consideration of the partial evidence about consequences can be informed by referring to epidemiological data. A very rough guide on outcomes is provided by data on death by motor vehicle traffic accidents in England and Wales (Office of Population Censuses and Surveys, 1993). Approximately 4,000 people die in motor vehicle accidents each year. However, we cannot assume from these data that it is always the driver who dies – this is frequently not the case – and so we cannot precisely calculate the risk associated with driving. And studying mortality ignores accidents that do not lead to death. With these caveats in mind, some generalizations can be made. Overall, men are nearly three times more likely than women to die in motor vehicle accidents. Women between 75 and 84 years of age are more than five times more likely to die in a motor vehicle traffic accident than women aged between 25 and 54. A man of the same age as my patient (75–84 group), or indeed a man aged between 15 and 24, both have a 70 per cent higher risk of dying in a motor vehicle traffic accident than a woman aged between 75 and 84. A man over 65 years of age is more than ten times as likely to die in a motor vehicle traffic accident than a woman between the ages of 25 and 54 (OPCS, 1993). Nevertheless, it is difficult to infer from these aggregated data and so determine which particular individuals, by reason of decreased performance or their attitude to risk taking, expose themselves and others to the risk of death or serious harm.

In this particular case, one approach might be for the doctor to inform the patient that they intended to write to the licensing authority suggesting that the patient undergo an independent assessment of her ability to drive. Although there are specific guidelines for doctors with regard to drivers with epilepsy, guidelines for doctors with regard to patients who are drivers and develop dementia are vague. Guidelines for medical practitioners propose, 'if early dementia, driving may be permitted if there is no significant disorientation in time and place, and there is adequate retention of insight and judgement. Annual medical review required' (Medical Advisory Branch DVLA, 1993). The word 'adequate' begs certain questions. It is difficult for doctors to assess the insight and judgement necessary to drive safely. And by the time patients are disorientated in time and place, they are likely to be severely demented and highly unsafe on the road.

In the light of the lack of evidence available it is difficult for doctors to know what to do, and so they must vary considerably in their judgement. If a doctor finds that a specific patient of my patient's age has been diagnosed as demented, what then is his or her responsibility? On the one hand, the doctor may say that it is the licensing authority's responsibility to re-test patients' performance at regular intervals as they get older. On the other hand, deaths have been reported as a consequence of patients with known but unreported Alzheimer's disease driving dangerously, for example, along a motorway in the wrong direction.

Deaths of these kinds could be avoided by GPs using their disease registers to identify demented patients with a view to preventing them from causing harm to themselves and others. This could even be a component of screening for the elderly. Tertiary prevention is the prevention of suffering and death consequent to known disease, so a programme of this kind might be seen as tertiary prevention at a national level. An obvious criticism of such a proposal is that it would involve a loss of trust between patients and doctors. Breaching confidentiality, which may undermine the doctor–patient relationship, might be sufficient to prevent some doctors from blowing the whistle on any patient. If doctors acted to protect the rest of the public systematically, some patients would be reluctant to come for health checks or confide their concerns about loss of memory and ability to function, for fear that this would result in further losses, such as the loss of their licence to drive.

There is a general distaste and rejection of anyone acting as a double agent and informing on a client's acts or omissions to another agency. This tale telling, fictionalized so well in *A Brave New World* (Huxley, 1959), is abhorrent to most people. And yet in other not too dissimilar situations, doctors are obliged to inform on their patients. Only one dental professional had been shown to have infected his patients with the HIV virus. But if doctors have other medical doctors as their patients and these refuse to follow advice in modifying their professional practice if they are found to be HIV positive, the responsible doctor is required to inform an appropriate regulatory body (General Medical Council, 1993). The risks to others of these doctors continuing to practise are probably considerably less than they are for a demented patient continuing to drive. More stringent criteria are therefore being applied in the medical profession's self-regulation regarding fitness to practise, and less respect is being given to confidential information than is the case for the general public.

Where legal obligations change or seem opaque, the need for an ethical framework which is separate from the law becomes more apparent. Doctors making difficult judgements need to take into account both medical ethics in terms of principles and consequences, and the current state of the law on an issue. Few doctors deliberately challenge the law on the grounds of ethical principles, as this requires considerable time, energy, resources and courage.

Doctors as prescribers

The second case described involved a patient who wanted me to prescribe drugs for infertility. I looked through her notes and found that approximately 1 year previously she had attended an NHS hospital and been fully investigated for her infertility. The specialists had concluded that she had suffered severe pelvic inflammatory disease in the past, and that the likelihood of her conceiving was so small that it did not justify proceeding with further therapy. The doctors had told the patient this, but had added that if she wanted further treatment they could suggest a local hospital where she could be seen privately.

One approach to the patient's request would be simply to copy the private prescription onto an NHS form and sign it. This would indicate respect for the patient's choice and would be likely to promote cordial relations between doctor and patient. A second approach to this request might be to explain the improbability of a successful conception to the patient and then ask her to decide what she wanted. A third approach might be to inform her of the high cost of the drugs and urge her, if she wanted the drug, to take her private prescription to the chemist and pay for it herself. Assuming that NHS resources are scarce and that their use in one area deprives other patients of care, this patient's continued attempts at pregnancy could prevent several other patients from receiving necessary treatments. This approach respects the patient's autonomy, but it weighs up this patient's needs against notions of opportunity costs and justice among patients. This explicit acknowledgement of scarce resources and the role of doctors in allocating resources has been urged by economists (McGuire, 1986) but it worries many doctors.

During the 1980s, the Department of Health became increasingly aware that District Health Authorities were transferring the responsibility for prescribing for NHS hospital out-patients to general practitioners in order to reduce their drug costs. Because of this trend, doctors were reminded that, 'the duty of prescribing for a particular element of a patient's treatment rests with the doctor who at the time had clinical responsibility for that element' (Peach, 1987). The decision as to which doctor has clinical responsibility for any particular aspect of a patient's treatment at any given time was 'for the doctors concerned to take'. This statement of policy is not particularly clear. The guidelines were restated, not because of the comparatively small cost of GPs copying private prescriptions onto

FP10s, but rather because of the considerable transferred cost of shifting prescribing from hospital out-patients to general practitioners.

One response to the patient's request would be to comply with her wish for an NHS prescription; this would respect the patient's wish for treatment. However, information about the high cost of the drugs might lead the doctor to be concerned about the opportunity costs or opportunities foregone in terms of other patients' needs, which would be sacrificed by doing what the patient wanted. This concern might be explicit if the doctor was a fundholder, and even a non-fundholder might be concerned that an excessive burden was being placed on tax payers for what was likely to be a placebo effect. Resources are finite and scarce in the NHS, but in spite of this the principle of justice is extremely difficult to apply in practice.

In the long run, it may seem inappropriate for doctors to impose their own values, thereby individually prioritizing the health services that they allocate to patients, although this approach is actually being fostered by the current trend towards fundholding. A fairer system might be one in which society decides, in advance of individuals having specific needs, about the priorities it will give to particular health services. This borrows from Rawls's (1971) idea of a contract being made about resource allocation in advance, without people knowing what will happen to them or what their needs will be in the future. Decisions about competing priorities could be made in the light of information about effectiveness provided by the medical profession. With a social consensus approach, the government, as purse-holder, could direct doctors to provide all the services to be made available within the budget allocated. Doctors would cease to decide individually about who should receive particular services, and they would also become immune from complaints about not providing services not covered by the programme.

This approach has been adopted in America by the state of Oregon (Kitzhaber, 1993). When obstetrical and gynaecological procedures were listed in terms of the order in which community representatives valued them, infertility services ranked second to bottom. With a limited budget they would not be funded by the programme (Kirk, 1993). This is an example of an approach which develops a social consensus about a policy which will determine how scarce public resources are to be allocated. It can be criticized for reducing the autonomy given to individuals and doctors to decide what to do about a particular condition, but it does this in order to provide resources for an agreed group of conditions which are available to all.

In summary, in a position of imperfect knowledge, moral principles help doctors reason and advise about decision-making in a more rigorous and defensible way. Knowledge about the probable consequences of actions will help doctors and patients to choose between different options. Patients who are well informed about benefits and harms are generally in the best position to decide about their own particular lives. For this reason, autonomy is generally considered to be fundamental. In a society which accepts that medical care is often too costly for those in need to pay for it, decisions about who pays, what should be paid for, and according to which criteria, will continue to be subjects for debate. Patients, doctors, the government, ethicists and economists are all legitimate and expert contributors to this debate.

References

Beauchamp, T. L. & Childress, J. F. (1983) *Principles of Biomedical Ethics*. New York: Oxford University Press.
General Medical Council (1993) *HIV Infection and AIDs: The Ethical Considerations*. London: GMC Circular.
Gillon, R. (1986) *Philosophical Medical Ethics*. Chichester: Wiley.
Huxley, A. (1959) *A Brave New World*. London: Chatto and Windus.
Kirk, E. P. (1993) The women's health care component of the Oregon Basic Health Care Plan. *American Journal of Obstetrics and Gynecology 168*: 1870–1874.
Kitzhaber, J. A. (1993) Rationing in action: Prioritizing health services in an era of limits: The Oregon experience. *British Medical Journal 307*: 373–377.
McGuire, A. (1986) Ethics and resource allocation: An economist's view. *Social Sciences and Medicine 22*: 1167–1174.
Medical Advisory Branch DVLA (1993) *For Medical Practitioners: At a Glance Guide to the Current Medical Standards of Fitness to Drive*. Swansea: DVLA.
Office of Population Censuses and Surveys (1993) *Mortality Statistics 1991. Causes*. London: HMSO.
Peach, L. (1987) *Prescribing Responsibility*. Letter DA (87) 10. London: Department of Health and Social Security.
Rawls, J. A. (1971) *A Theory of Justice*. Cambridge: Harvard University Press, Massachusetts.
Russell, B. (1984) *A History of Western Philosophy*, 2nd edn. London: Counterpoint, Unwin Paperbacks.
Scambler, G. (1989) *Epilepsy*. London: Tavistock/Routledge.
Scruton, R. (1982) *Kant*. Oxford: Oxford University Press.

9

The Economic Aspects of General Practice

> Mr Mettle was a 59-year-old lorry driver. He came to see me because he had back pain which was making it difficult for him to drive for long periods. I arranged some physiotherapy. When I next saw him I found that he had a slight foot-drop, and I referred him to a local orthopaedic surgeon. The surgeon initially managed the problem conservatively, and then booked the patient for surgery, which was performed approximately a year later. After this, the patient's condition was unchanged and he took early retirement.

> Mr Blunt was a 35-year-old policeman complaining of back pain. He had no neurological signs, but as he was concerned about the implications of his condition on his work and had private medical insurance, I referred him to a specialist. He underwent a discectomy the following week. He continued to have pain after the operation and it took about a year of rehabilitation before he could go back to work.

Introduction

These two cases raise many issues about effectiveness, efficiency and access to medical care. Some people have taken a rather romantic view of resource allocation and demanded that the government provide all that they consider necessary to meet medical 'needs'. An introduction to economic issues is not provided in medical schools, even though the provision of medical care is the largest industry or service in the country, accounting for more than 5 per cent of national expenditure or 10 per cent of taxpayers' money. Refusal to learn the language of economics and engage in an adult dialogue with those who are responsible for resource allocation may reflect feelings of professional pride and a distaste for money and trade, but it also puts doctors, nurses and patients at a profound disadvantage. Not understanding or contributing to the debate about resource allocation may contribute to the low political evaluation of the health service when measured in terms of the resources allocated to it. The Organization for Economic Co-operation and Development (OECD) has reviewed systems of financing health and expenditure in seven European countries (1992) and found that the United Kingdom's expenditure on health as a percentage share of gross domestic product was the lowest, at 6.2 per cent, of any of the seven countries examined. This low national expenditure on medical care may be seen as a success by some, and as a failure by others.

The aim of this chapter is to introduce ideas and evidence about the uses of economics. At the present time, economic theory with regard to the provision of medical care is still at an early stage of development, but, given that resources are scarce, it seems reasonable and appropriate for policy makers to design a mixture of incentives in order to deliver an optimum volume and mix of medical care, with optimum access to services, at the least cost possible.

Economic theories

The first step, it seems to me, when learning from successes or failures, is to be able to think and talk about them. Doctors are the main decision-makers when it comes to allocating resources within the health service, and economists have tried to erect plausible models to explain their behaviours. Tussing (1985) suggested three motivational systems. The first is the agency model, in which the doctor supplies technical expertise and acts solely in the interests of the patient. When the service involves the patient in out-of-pocket payments, this model includes helping the patient to choose treatments which balance the likely benefits of care against the likely cost. The second model is the self-interest model, in which the doctor is motivated significantly by the desire to maximize some combination of his or her income and leisure. The third is the medical ethics model, where the doctor is motivated primarily by the desire to do as much as possible for the individual patient at hand, irrespective of the cost. The first and third motivational systems have been discussed in the chapter on medical ethics. In this context, it is perhaps worth noting that economics developed as a discipline in association with ethics in departments of philosophy. Economists from Adam Smith to Maynard Keynes saw themselves as concerned jointly with ethics and economics, and these subjects need not be construed as being polar opposites. The discussion in this chapter is based on the assumption that doctors are driven by a mixture of motives, and that the quality of their behaviour and the adequacy of the system depends partly on successfully harnessing professional self-interest with society's objectives.

Before considering the evidence about the way in which doctors' financial self-interest affects the functioning of the system, some concepts need to be clarified. Upon examination of most markets, a clear product can be identified. However, this is not the case in medicine. Whereas a new car or a new book may provide direct satisfaction to the consumer, medical care rarely provides direct satisfaction. Evans (1984) pointed out that the immediate effect of most medical care, for example, dentistry, drugs, diagnostic and therapeutic interventions and hospital stays, is negative; they are uncomfortable, even frightening. Consumption of most medical care is a negative experience and not something that consumers seek willingly, even if they have private medical insurance or a service guaranteed to be free at the point of use. It is quite difficult to think of a medical act, the consumption of which brings anyone direct satisfaction, although, interestingly, it may be that it is more likely to be found in primary care. For example, an anxious patient who phones for reassurance about a sick child at night may state that this reassurance has brought them great relief. This notwithstanding, doctors who have also had experience as patients will recognize that this process is generally uncomfortable.

Medical care also differs from other commodities because it is perceived to have a mediating role in enabling the consumer or patient to achieve better health. Recognition of this mediating role

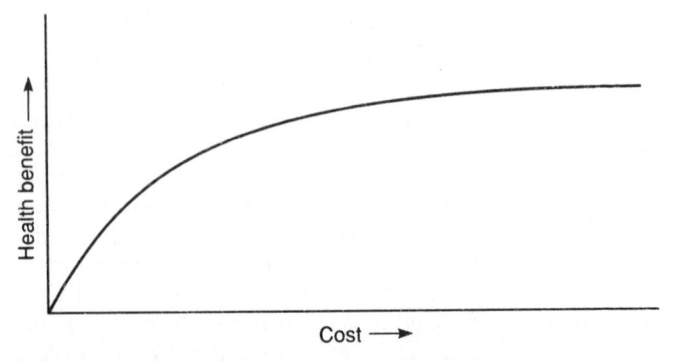

Fig. 9.1 Diminishing marginal returns. (From Enthoven, 1980).

is important for an understanding of the concept of under and over-utilization. Under-utilization implies there are amounts and types of care which are not supplied and which, if available, could increase the health status of some patients. Over-utilization implies that patients are receiving something to a greater degree than can reasonably be judged to do them any good. This concept of benefits or outcomes links up with medical ethics and epidemiology. Enthoven (1980) described the relationship between health status and the expenditure of resources on manpower, capital and raw materials. He suggested that it was likely that up to a certain point the allocation of resources would improve health status. However, he also pointed out that it was possible that in some circumstances more resources would not lead to improved health status. He described this as 'flat-of-the-curve' medicine. This is an example of the law of diminishing marginal returns, a basic principle of economics. It is illustrated in Figure 9.1.

Illich (1976) and Stoate (1989) have suggested that additional resource allocation in some areas of health care may actually be hazardous to health. For example, more Caesarean sections, tonsillectomies or screening may lead to risk without benefit, and could reasonably be regarded as over-utilization.

A problem here is that each doctor, whether providing specialist or primary care, may act with the best of intentions, but with imperfect information, and so be highly resistant to the suggestion that the curve is flat for the services they provide. These ideas have been posed by the economists Enthoven (1980) and Evans (1984), but the uncertainty about the outcomes to which they allude was also a problem identified by the epidemiologist Cochrane (1972). One popular theory in British medicine is that the government is stingy, rather than that resources are scarce. A second popular theory is that there is a direct relationship between the level of medical activity and beneficial outcomes for patients. The limited effect overall of the process of medical care on health status generally is puzzling. Part of the puzzle can be explained, as McKeown (1979) and others have done, by drawing attention to the much more powerful influence that socio-economic factors have on health and illness. The process of medical care was, and still is, comparatively powerless in reducing the adverse effect of lifestyle influences on health and life expectancy.

Cochrane (1972) pointed out that practitioners were fairly resistant to making rigorous observations about the natural history of disease in a prospective way. He stressed the importance of testing medical interventions through randomized control trials. When medical scientists have not provided information about the effectiveness of resources allocated to one form of activity or another, it is difficult for economists to make recommendations about the efficient allocation of resources. What is the appropriate level of Caesarean sections or tonsillectomies? Does it matter if there is a long waiting list for the insertion of gromets? Until the medical specialist can provide evidence about what is and is not effective, it is difficult to know how money should best be spent. The type and level of expenditure should of course depend on the results of controlled trials and comparisons of different treatments and outcomes. When the average consumer intends to buy a new microwave, he or she may go to the local library and weigh up the relative costs and benefits by referring to a consumer's guide. In the case of expensive and sometimes vital medical treatments, it therefore seems remarkable that this kind of information is often not considered worth the cost and effort needed to produce it.

Economic evidence

Having started by considering the general issues and problems arising when approaching medical care from an economic perspective, a second challenge is to analyze the evidence which suggests that the volume and style with which medical care is delivered is, partially at least, determined by doctors' desires to maximize some combination of their own income and leisure. It is always easier to spot self-interest in others, and so I will start by considering some evidence about the delivery of secondary care. The general practitioner's simultaneous roles as advocate and gate-keeper makes an understanding of this relevant when weighing up the relative advantages and disadvantages of accepting the status quo against changes in national policy and finance. One way to examine the possible association between economic incentives and behaviour is to compare and contrast methods of remuneration for doctors in different countries and the services provided for patients. Bunker (1970) and Vayda (1973) et al. (1982) compared and contrasted the health care systems of North America with those of Britain. Bunker found that there were twice as many surgeons in the United States per head of population, and that they were reimbursed on a fee-for-services basis. He found that when the rate of elective surgery, like cholecystectomy, tonsillectomy and haemorrhoidectomy, was compared in the United States and the United Kingdom, two to three times as many operations were performed per head of population in the United States. However, when non-elective or less elective surgery, for example, thyroidectomy rates were compared, there was much less difference between North America and Britain. Vayda obtained similar calculations for the United States, Canada and the United Kingdom. He found the highest rate of elective surgery in the United States, followed by Canada and then the

United Kingdom. Physicians and surgeons in the United States and Canada are both remunerated on a fee-for-service basis, whereas in Britain they are paid on a salaried basis for their NHS work. Vayda found particularly large differences in the cholecystectomy rate; these were performed five times more frequently in North America.

Speculating on the reasons for these differences, Culyer and others (1981, 1982) pointed out that in the United States, where only part of the population is insured for health care, some patients are under-serviced and these individuals are particularly likely to be the uninsured. In contrast, insured people have no disincentive to seek care regardless of the cost, and their doctors may tend to compete for reduced overall demand by generating extra demand for services among this group. This combination of motivation and behaviour may lead to a higher elective intervention rate. These kinds of comparisons do not of course answer the basic epidemiological question as to what an optimum level of surgery might be, nor is it clear that North American doctors are acting entirely out of self-interest, or in a way that implicitly conflicts with the best interests of their patients. Their norms for operating are much higher, and these may be considered to represent good practice. Bunker *et al.* (1974) found that physicians in the United States submitted themselves to elective surgery as frequently as other professional groups, and physicians' wives underwent significantly more surgical procedures like cholecystectomy and hysterectomy than the wives of other professionals.

Enthoven (1985, 1986), an American economist, visited Britain and appraised the problems of the National Health Service in documents that have had a profound effect on the language, thought and policy of health service managers. Enthoven identified large spending differences between the United States and the United Kingdom. The United States, at that time, were spending about 11 per cent of their gross national product on health care, compared with about 5.5 per cent in the United Kingdom. Enthoven made it clear that neither government would wish to see costs increase. Within this context, he identified the major challenge for the NHS as being a need to achieve good performance through 'real incentives' rather than relying on dedication and idealism.

The first problem Enthoven identified concerned consultants and their waiting lists. In the 1980s, NHS consultants were paid by salary and they had long-term contracts with the NHS. Enthoven wrote, 'I'm told most consultants say to their patients, "You need the operation; it will take place sometime in the next year or so, and we'll call you a week in advance to tell you when to come into hospital".' He said this practice reinforced the authority and status of the consultant, and 'embarrassingly', the length of a consultant's

NHS waiting list. This in turn created a demand for his services from private patients. Clearing a waiting list was directly opposed to the economic interest of the consultant. This problem is illustrated by the two cases of back pain which I observed and which were managed quite differently.

It is by now well known that Enthoven proposed 'an internal market' as a solution to this problem. He then went back to America. Putting these recommendations into practice without increased resources is an ongoing process. The relationship between theory and practice in economics is as problematic as it is elsewhere, and, just as is true for doctors, it is never clear whether economists' prescriptions provide solutions or create new problems.

Having identified a relationship between the system of financing and the behaviour of doctors in the secondary care sector, let us now consider the primary care sector. Little research has been done in this area, but there is some evidence from both sides of the Atlantic that financial considerations do have some effect on the service provided for patients. Hemenway *et al.* (1990) examined the role of doctors in a major chain of ambulatory care centres operating for profit in the United States. Initially, the physicians were paid a flat hourly wage. However, in 1985 the doctors were offered extra bonuses, the size of which depended on the gross incomes they generated individually by requesting laboratory tests, return visits and so on. The practice patterns of 15 doctors were compared before and after the new incentive scheme. Thirteen of the 15 doctors ordered more laboratory tests per visit, and as a group the 15 doctors ordered 23 per cent more tests per visit. In the one-year period analyzed, the number of office visits per month increased by 12 per cent, average charges per visit increased by 15 per cent, and the total charges per month increased by 28 per cent. The wages of the seven physicians who regularly earned a bonus rose by 19 per cent. The investigators concluded that substantial monetary incentives based on individual performance may induce a group of physicians to increase the intensity of their practice, even though not all of them benefited from the incentives. This may seem a far cry from the NHS, and it is perhaps too soon to measure the effects of the new system of incentives imposed by the 1990 Health Service Act. However, there is some evidence of an increase in the provision of those tests which are financially rewarded, such as cervical screening (Reid *et al.*, 1991).

What evidence is there that the remuneration system in Britain affects the style of health care delivery to patients in general practice? Calnan *et al.* (1992) reviewed the evidence collected in their workload study. They postulated that in capitation systems the total number of hours worked by GPs would be likely to be relatively unaffected by higher patient load. A higher patient load might typically be managed by seeing more patients in the same time period. In other words, GPs would have a tendency not to increase the number of hours worked in proportion to an increase in list size. Analyzing their survey data, Calnan *et al.* found that there was an inverse linear relationship between list size and booking interval. This evidence was derived before the new contract when capitation accounted for only about 45 per cent of GPs' incomes. The restructuring of the NHS in the early 1990s involved increasing the proportion of remuneration for GPs which depended on their list size. There had previously been a gradual trend towards reduced list size and increased booking intervals. It remains to be seen to what extent changing economic incentives will reverse or at least arrest the trend towards longer consultations.

Enthoven (1985) also deprecated the lack of incentives for GPs to reduce the number of referrals and to prescribe economically. Incentives for both these practices are now in operation for fundholders. It is not yet clear to what extent they will change doctors' behaviour in the long run.

The social context

It is difficult for economists, just as it is for doctors, to divorce their theories from their own particular cultural and historical traditions. This problem was highlighted by the Chicago economist Friedman (1985) when he was asked to reflect on the work of the influential Cambridge economist, Keynes. Friedman explained why Keynes was able to develop an economic theory in Britain in the early twentieth century which was fundamentally different from the theory Friedman developed in the United States after the Second World War.

Friedman said that in Britain at the time Keynes developed his ideas, there was a spirit of *noblesse oblige*. The government and civil service were by and large able, benevolent and incorruptible. In this context, Keynes' vision of economists acting to engineer preferred outcomes, for example, full employment, was perceived to be both benevolent and realistic. Friedman argued that the situation was entirely different in the United States. There was no tradition of an incorruptible or able civil service, and public attitudes focused on self-interest and the spoils system. In this context, it seemed logical and realistic for Friedman to develop a theory, sometimes called the market model, from an economic theory which was popular in Britain before the era of benign government interventionism and Keynesian economics.

It may seem something of a paradox that it was an American economist, Enthoven, who subsequently popularized the language and the application of the market model for the British health service in the belief that dedication and idealism were 'old hat'. Enthoven observed that the American market system cost more, but paradoxically advocated a market system to achieve increased efficiency in Britain. Titmuss (1970) had argued conversely that harnessing altruistic as well as other forces made the British medical care system work more efficiently. If altruism is not named and valued by economists, will it disappear? Changes in the NHS cannot be evaluated independently from other factors like patients' expectations and economic cycles like boom and recession which are also changing. It will therefore be difficult to evaluate the result of changing the economic language and incentives in the British system.

Evans (1984) quoted a Cambridge economist, Joan Robinson, who said, 'We study economics, not to understand the economy, but to avoid being deceived by economists'. Robinson was making a point about her own profession, with its particular assumptions and framework which may guide or mislead others. The same point could be made for any discipline which has its own jargon and mystique, like philosophy or medicine. Robinson was trying to highlight the importance of theory or language. She would probably concede that it is also important to study economics in order to enter into the debate, and to understand the economy too.

References

Bunker, J. R. (1970) Surgical manpower: A comparison of operations and surgeons in the United States and in England and Wales. *New England Journal of Medicine* 282: 135–144.

Bunker, J. P., Byron, B. M. & Brown, B. W. (1974) The physician-patient as an informed consumer of surgical services. *New England Journal of Medicine* 290: 1051–1055.

Calnan, M., Groenewegen, P. P. & Hutten, J. (1992) Professional reimbursement and management of time in general practice: An international comparison. *Social Science and Medicine* 35: 207–216.

Cochrane, A. L. (1972) *Effectiveness and Efficiency. Random Reflections on Health Services*. London: Nuffield Provincial Hospitals Trust.

Culyer, A. J. (1982) The NHS and the market: Images and realities. In: McLachlan & Maynard, A. (eds) *The Public/Private Mix for Health*. London: Nuffield Provincial Hospitals Trust.

Culyer, A. J., Maynard, A. & Williams, A. (1981) Alternative systems of health care provision: An essay on motes and beams. In: Olson, M. (ed.) *A New Approach to the Economics of Health Care*. Washington DC: American Enterprise for Public Policy Research.

Enthoven, A. C. (1980) *Health Plan: The Only Practical Solution to the Soaring Cost of Medical Care*. Reading, Massachusetts: Addison-Wesley.

Enthoven, A. C. (1985) *Reflections on the Management of the National Health Service: An American Looks at Incentives to Efficiency in Health Services Management in the UK*. London: Nuffield Provincial Hospitals Trust.

Enthoven, A. C. (1986) National Health Service: Some reforms that might be politically feasible. *The Economist 22 June:* 61–64.

Evans, R. G. (1984) *Strained Mercy: The Economics of Canadian Health Care*. Toronto: Butterworth.

Friedman, M. (1985) Keynes's political legacy In: Burton, J. (ed.) *Keynes' General Theory 50 Years On*. London: Institute of Economic Affairs.

Hemenway, D., Killen, A., Cashman, S., Parks, C. L. & Bicknell, W. J. (1990) Physicians' responses to financial incentives: Evidence from a for-profit ambulatory care centre. *New England Journal of Medicine 322:* 1059–1063.

Illich, I. (1976) *Limits to Medicine; Medical Nemesis: The Expropriation of Health*. Middlesex: Penguin Books Ltd.

McKeown, T. (1979) *The Role of Medicine: Dream, Mirage or Nemesis?* Oxford: Blackwell Publishers Ltd.

OECD (1992) The reform of health care systems: a comparative analysis of 7 OECD countries. *Health Policy Studies*, no. 2. Paris: OECD.

Reid, G. S., Robertson, A. J., Bisset, C., Smith, J., Waugh, N. & Halkerston, R. (1991) Cervical screening in Perth and Kinross since introduction of the new contract. *British Medical Journal 303:* 447–450.

Stoate, H. G. (1989) Can health screening damage your health? *Journal of the Royal College of General Practitioners 39:* 193–195.

Titmuss, R. (1970) *The Gift Relationship: From Human Blood to Social Policy*. London: George Allen and Unwin Ltd.

Tussing, A. D. (1985) *Irish Medical Care Resources: An Economic Analysis*, paper 126. Dublin: The Economic and Social Research Institute.

Vayda, E. (1973) A comparison of surgical rates in Canada and in England and Wales. *New England Journal of Medicine 289:* 1224–1230.

Vayda, E., Mindell, W. R. & Rutkow, I. M. (1982) A decade of surgery in Canada, England and Wales, and the United States. *Archives of Surgery 117:* 846–853.

10
Making Sense of Workload Studies

> 'Picture a middle-aged man who has not troubled to keep up with developments in his continuously changing profession since he qualified 20 years ago. He sees clients for two or three brief periods each week, spending the rest of his time on the golf course.'
>
> (Anon)
> *The Economist*, 1987

> 'GPs in the United Kingdom devote the least amount of time to the provision of care, 38.2 hours a week, compared with more than 50 hours for GPs in France and the United States.'
>
> (Sandier)
> *Organization for Economic Co-operation and Development*, 1990

Introduction

These passages appeared in an *Economist* editorial titled 'Let doctors compete: Britain's general practitioners need a new prescription', and in an OECD review by Sandier of the work and income of doctors, which was based on data provided by the Department of Health and Social Security (DHSS, 1987). The image of the GP on the golf course is a tenacious one. It may have had some element of truth at some period, for some doctors. Surveys of workload have added figures to a confusing array of different terms. The difference between image, apparently neutral statistics and my own personal experience posed a challenge. The aim of this chapter is to analyze the terminology and the evidence used in the debate about GPs work load.

In the 1980s, general practitioners in the NHS contracted to provide patient care continuously for 168 hours each week (DOH, 1989). Four years after the DOH survey cited by the OECD, the DOH undertook a second workload study (DOH, 1991). These figures will be examined because they are more recent, but they do not differ substantially from the results of the first survey (DHSS, 1987). It is difficult to measure what GPs do. The DOH sent structured diaries to GPs to fill in for one week. A predetermined number of doctors were sent the diary during each week of the year which was surveyed. The working week of the sample of GPs who responded was apportioned according to different categories. Inferring from this sample, an estimate was then made of the work performed by GPs generally.

Extrapolating from the sample of GPs who responded, about 5 per cent of doctors worked and remained on call for 130–168 hours per week, but most GPs worked less than the contract implied. Ninety per cent of doctors worked between 30 and 130 hours a week, and 5 per cent of doctors worked less than 30 hours a week. What accounts for the difference between these figures and those quoted in the OECD summary?

What was counted and discounted in the figure for hours worked?

The 38 or 37 hours counted in the first and second studies (DHSS, 1987; DOH, 1991) included seeing patients in surgery, clinics and at home, and it also included practice administration, case discussion and paperwork. It excluded attendance at educational courses and at advisory committees, such as local medical committees (LMCs) and District Health Authorities (DHAs). It also excluded teaching medical students, hospital appointments and research. When the hours spent on these and other 'non-general medical services' were averaged, they amounted to 5 additional hours per week. When this is included, the average GP worked a more respectable 42 daytime hours per week.

A second exclusion from the DOH summary figure was time spent on call at night and at the weekend. Salisbury (1993) demonstrated a rising trend of patient demand for service during the night between 1982 and 1992, with an increase in night visit claims of 39 per cent during this period. Sutherland and Cooper (1992) found increased stress was reported by doctors as a result of night visits and telephone calls which interrupted family life. When doctors actually made a visit, this was counted as work. But in the DOH workload study, an additional 23 hours on average were spent by doctors on call at night or at the weekend. This time could certainly not be regarded as free time or free of stress. When this is included, time spent working or on call amounted to 65 hours per week, a figure which is quite different from the summary figure of 37 hours which was, and still is, quoted.

What was counted in the denominator?

In the DOH Workload Survey (1991), the products 37, 42 and 65 hours worked per week were achieved by totalling the hours worked by doctors and dividing the figure produced by the total number of doctors. Reimbursement for cervical screening has drawn attention to the problem which is inherent in calculating averages in this way. The problem is that whatever the size of the numerator (women screened), the larger the denominator (or total population of women), the lower the product is likely to be. Taking the example of target percentage payments, a list size which is inflated by too many 'ghost' patients will result in a lower percentage reimbursement for smears undertaken. In the case of doctors' working hours, the denominator included doctors who were away on holiday or on sick leave. When these 'ghost' doctors were removed from the denominator when calculating average working hours, the figures rose to 41, 46 and 72 hours per week in each category.

Besides these 'ghosts', the denominator also contained a heterogeneous mixture of working people. Hooper *et al.* (1989) found that approximately half of women doctors worked part-time, and they received a lower share of the practice income in return. But if these doctors worked more than the minimum required to make them eligible for a full basic practice allowance, the DOH counted the hours they worked as if they were full-timers. This resulted in a decrease in the calculated average number of hours the 'average' GP worked, which was then wrongly assumed to represent full-time work.

The DOH found that the average woman spent 36 hours seeing patients, doing administrative and case discussion work, whereas the average man spent 42 hours on these activities. Osler (1991) found that approximately one-half of part-time women GPs did no general practice work at night and at the weekend. So it is likely that including these people in calculations of out-of-hours work brought this figure down even more.

At the time the study was undertaken, doctors did not have to retire at 70 years of age as they currently do. Many practitioners continued to work for many years beyond the usual retirement age. In addition, they claimed a pension, having taken '24-hour retirement'. Provided these GPs worked more than the minimum time required to be eligible for a full-time allowance, they were also counted as full-timers in the DOH statistics. These semi-retired doctors were found to have worked on average 34 hours per week. The concepts of full and part-time are difficult ones, in a profession where part-timers work as long as full-timers in other trades. But including the hours worked by these two types of part-timers when calculating full-timers' hours of work in general practice must have reduced the average numbers of hours worked by general practitioner full-timers considerably. And in most subsequent studies, the hours worked by part-timers have been included in workload calculations in the same way. Until these figures are excluded, there can be no accurate assessment of full-time work.

List size, workload and the time spent with patients on consultations

Butler and Calnan (1987, 1988) were funded by the DOH to make a cross-sectional study of the relationship between GPs' list size and workload. They found an association between list size and time spent with patients. Table 10.1 draws on Calnan and Butler's data (1988) to estimate the time spent on average per patient per year according to the list size of the doctor.

Table 10.1 *List size and average time spent per patient per year.*

Patient list size	Mean consultation time per annum (minutes)
<1,500	43
>3,000	20

The difference in the time doctors spent with patients was due to many factors, two important ones being that doctors with smaller lists on average provided longer consultations, and they saw their patients more frequently.

Many other factors are associated with the size of a doctor's list. Table 10.2 draws on Butler and Calnan's data to illustrate the different characteristics of GPs with large and small list sizes.

Table 10.2 Doctors' characteristics in relation to their average list size.

Patient list size	Male GPs (%)	Aged 46-65 years (%)	Rural GPs (%)
<1,500	53%	34%	23%
>3,000	90%	63%	4%

The DOH workload study findings can be used to complete a picture of how different list sizes relate to different practice activity. In 1989–90, the average GP provided 146 consultations per week, lasting on average 9 minutes each. The top one-third of GPs in terms of consultation activity saw from 150 to over 300 patients per week. The number of consultations doctors provided varied with list size. More than 50 per cent of doctors with a list size of over 3,500 provided 225 plus consultations in a week. Less than 5 per cent of doctors with a list size of less than 1,000 provided this many consultations. Workload studies have not documented the reasons for consultations from the point of view of patients' demands and needs.

One-quarter of the average doctor's consultations would probably have been for respiratory infections. It might have been appropriate to get through these swiftly, although the evidence about patients' beliefs and concerns presented in Chapter 4 may make this behaviour seem questionable. A quarter to a third of the week's consultations might have involved patients with symptoms of psychological distress. The average GP in the workload study may have seen 50 patients per week with psychological distress. But doctors with large list sizes might routinely have seen 100 patients per week with psychological distress. Butler and Calnan found doctors who had larger lists provided shorter consultations on average. Howie et al. (1991) found doctors who provided shorter consultations were less likely to identify psychosocial problems. This does not seem surprising when one considers the numbers of potential problems they might have uncovered. Doctors with large lists who attempted to identify psychosocial problems accurately would rapidly burn out.

Morrell and Roland (1987) suggested an average of 10 minutes per consultation allowed time for high quality care. They proposed that in order to create sufficient time available for longer consultations, smaller list sizes of on average 1,750 would be needed, and perhaps even smaller numbers in areas of high demand and high need. Butler and Calnan's evidence supports the thesis that smaller list size was associated with more time spent with patients, but it was also clear from their data that the characteristics of GPs with different list sizes were different. It is difficult to extrapolate from a cross-sectional study about cause and effect. However, the DOH studies have been repeated several times. This does not provide a longitudinal picture, but where the same definitions were used, it does provide a series of cross-sectional views. The DOH (1991) found that between 1985–6 and 1989–90, the total number of GPs had risen by approximately 1,500, and the time spent on consultations had increased significantly too. Many other factors changed during this period, such as an increase in women doctors, so inferences about cause and effect must be tentative.

Different patients and different consultation times: the consumer demand side of the equation

Many factors create a 'demand pull' for the supply of consultation time. Preston-Whyte and colleagues (1983) looked at the effect of a principal's gender on consultation patterns. Women patients preferred to consult women GPs, especially for smears, contraception other than 'the Pill' and gynaecological problems. Buchan and Richardson (1973) found the most time-consuming physical examination was the vaginal examination. This took over 3 minutes on average, three times longer than is usually spent examining the patient. There is also evidence that patients of either sex with psychological problems are more likely to consult female doctors (Marks et al., 1979; Boardman, 1987). And such consultations take longer (Raynes and Cairns, 1980). Women and those with psychological problems are known to consult more frequently (RCGP, OPCS, DHSS, 1986). These are all patient demand influences which might lead women doctors to provide longer and more frequent consultations.

Balarajan et al. (1992) examined the effect on GP workload created by economic deprivation. The investigators used data provided by patients about their consultations for the General Household Survey which is conducted by the Office of Population Censuses and Surveys annually. From these self-report data, they found that patients who lived in council accommodation consulted GPs significantly more frequently than patients who were owner-occupiers. Those who did not have access to a car consulted more frequently than patients who had access to transport by car. And adults born in New Commonwealth countries or Pakistan consulted more frequently than adults born in the United Kingdom.

Balarajan et al. (1992) estimated that a GP with an average list size of 2,000 in Spitalfields, for example, would receive 1,135 more consultations than the national average per year, whereas a GP working in South Cheam would have 503 fewer consultations. Le Grand (1978) and Townsend and Davidson (1982) found the demand for consultations expressed by groups who are relatively economically deprived may actually understate their extra need for medical care in terms of increased morbidity and mortality. In other words, those who are economically deprived may consult more frequently but still receive less care for equivalent levels of ill-health. So doctors in deprived areas are likely to see their patients more frequently and still perceive more unmet needs than doctors working in more economically privileged areas.

The pay for the job

Workload studies have tended to focus only on hours worked rather than the income–work package. This may have been partially because the DOH studies provided data which were used for the doctors' pay review, and because investigators wanted to avoid circular thinking. Researchers may also have feared that questions about income would reduce doctors' willingness to respond or the reliability of the data. From a political standpoint, it may also have been because doctors' pay negotiators have been less concerned with the fact that estimates of work and income include part-timers, as this would have resulted in an understatement of the income of full-timers. But surveys by Leese and Bosanquet (1989) and Hooper (1989) suggest that doctors are willing to provide information about income, and that income varies a great deal.

The main focus of Bosanquet and Leese's study was on differences between doctors with regard to innovative practice; this will be presented in Chapter 11. These researchers were able to show that within the same area, innovative practices generally earned more. But they also found that doctors in some areas, like the Thames Valley and eastern rural areas earned more on average than doctors in inner-city London or the urban Midlands. This was especially the case if they were innovative and/or dispensing practices. These area/dispensing differences in income were so large that doctors in inner-city London, even if they were innovative, earned less on average than doctors working in eastern rural areas who had not been innovative. These differences, derived from cross-sectional survey work, cannot be explained easily. They are likely to be the result of complex social and economic forces. However, they do at least suggest that income is not evenly distributed among GPs, and that the differences cannot necessarily be explained by GPs' style of work. A picture may be emerging of economically more privileged doctors working with economically more privileged patients. And current government policy may make these differences more marked.

A second major difficulty in making sense of the work–income package is in calculating what is, or should be, the income of those who work less than full time; these are generally, although not exclusively, women. Hooper (1989) found that approximately one-half of the women GPs who responded to a survey received a maximum or full share of practice profits. This implied that the agreement reached after negotiation within each group practice was that these doctors contributed hours equivalent to those worked by full-time partners. Hooper *et al.* (1989) reported that one-half of women GPs received less than a full-time partner's income and worked fewer hours. The investigators found dissatisfaction with earnings among part-time GPs. This may have reflected a lack of consensus within groups about the share of profits which should be attached to longer hours and night and weekend work.

Osler (1991) subsequently looked at the employment experiences of doctors who had trained in the early 1980s. She found that full-timers, either men or women, felt that their earnings were fair relative to their work. But fewer than half of the part-time profit-sharing partners reported that their pay was proportional to their work. Estimating fair shares must have been difficult for the doctors in the practices, and it is also difficult for investigators who intend to measure the consequences of intra-practice negotiations. In Osler's study, approximately one-half of part-timers worked both during the normal working day and at nights and weekends, but with reduced hours, while the other half worked during normal working hours and had no out-of-hours commitments. In the first group the average daytime workload was estimated as 73 per cent of that of a full-timer's, and the average out-of-hours work was estimated as 61 per cent. The mean percentage of the full profit share received by them was 55 per cent. The group that did not work out of hours were estimated to work on average 71 per cent of the daytime work of a full-timer, and to receive a mean 42 per cent of a full profit share. These figures are based on self-reports.

The work of Leese and Bosanquet (1989), Hooper (1989) and Osler (1991) questions assumptions about fairness in the distribution of work and income among doctors. National studies are needed to address these issues. Without information of this kind, policy makers in the government and the medical profession are perpetuating ignorance, and possibly a double standard, whereby an underclass of doctors may work more for less pay. There may be a process for doctors whereby 'winners' choose where they will practise, lead professional groups and negotiate income from a strong position. A process of self-selection within the medical profession may mirror and perpetuate Tudor Hart's 'inverse care' law, so that practices and doctors who need more resources actually get less.

References

Anon (1987) Let doctors compete: Britain's general practitioners need a new prescription. *The Economist,* November 21: 19–20.

Balarajan, R., Yuen, P. & Machin, D. (1992) Deprivation and the general practitioner workload. *British Medical Journal* 304: 529–534.

Boardman, A. P. (1987) The General Health Questionnaire and the detection of emotional disorders by general practitioners. *British Journal of Psychiatry* 151: 373–381.

Buchan, I. C. & Richardson, I. M. (1973) *Time Study of Consultations in General Practice.* Scottish Health Service Studies, no. 27. Edinburgh: Scottish Home and Health Department.

Butler, J. R. & Calnan, M. W. (1987) List sizes and use of time in general practice. *British Medical Journal* 295: 1383–1386.

Butler, J. R. & Calnan, M. W. (1988) *Too Many Patients? A Study of the Economy of Time and Standards of Care in General Practice.* Aldershot: Gower Publishing.

Calnan, M. & Butler, J. R. (1988) The economy of time in general practice: an assessment of the influence of list size. *Social Science and Medicine* 26: 435–441.

Department of Health (1989) *Terms of Service for Doctors in General Practice.* Crown Copyright.

Department of Health (1991) *General Medical Practitioners Workload (Survey 1989–1990). A Report Prepared for the Doctors' and Dentists' Review Body.* London: DOH.

Department of Health and Social Security (1987) *General Medical Practitioners Workload. A Report Prepared for the Doctors' and Dentists' Review Body (1985/1986).* London: DHSS.

Hooper, J. (1989) Full-time women general practitioners – an invaluable asset. *Journal of the Royal College of General Practitioners* 39: 289–291.

Hooper, J., Millar, J., Schofield, P. & Ward, G. (1989) Part-time women general practitioners – workload and remuneration. *Journal of the Royal College of General Practitioners* 39: 400–403.

Howie, J. G. R., Porter, A. M. D., Heaney, D. J. & Hopton, J. L. (1991) Long to short consultation ratio: A proxy measure of quality of care for general practice. *British Journal of General Practice* 41: 48–54.

Leese, B. & Bosanquet, N. (1989) High and low incomes in general practice. *British Medical Journal* 298: 932–934.

Le Grand, J. (1978) The distribution of public expenditure: The case for health care. *Economica* 45: 125–142.

Marks, J. N., Goldberg, D. P. & Hillier, V. F. (1979) Determinants of the ability of general practitioners to detect psychiatric illness. *Psychological Medicine* 9: 337–353.

Morrell, D. C. & Roland, M. O. (1987) How can good general practitioner care be achieved? *British Medical Journal* 294: 161–162.

Osler, K. (1991) Employment experiences of vocationally trained doctors. *British Medical Journal* 303: 762–764.

Preston-Whyte, M. E., Fraser, R. C. & Beckett, J. L. (1983) Effect of a principal's gender on consultation patterns. *Journal of the Royal College of General Practitioners* 33: 654–658.

Raynes, N. V. & Cairns, V. (1980) Factors contributing to the length of general practice consultations. *Journal of the Royal College of General Practitioners* 30: 496–498.

Royal College of General Practitioners, Office of Population Censuses and Surveys, Department of Health and Social Security (1981/1982) (1986) *Morbidity Statistics from General Practice – Third National Study*. London: HMSO 1986.

Salisbury, C. (1993) Visiting through the night. *British Medical Journal* 306: 762–764.

Sandier, S. (1990) Health services utilization and physician income trends. In: *Organization for Economic Co-operation and Development Health Care Systems in Transition: The Search for Efficiency*. Paris: OECD.

Sutherland, V. J. & Cooper, C. L. (1992) Job stress, satisfaction and mental health among general practitioners before and after introduction of the new contract. *British Medical Journal* 304: 1545–1548.

Townsend, P. & Davidson, N. (1982) *Inequalities in Health: The Black Report*. London: Penguin Books.

11
Diffusion of Innovation

> The community in which I practise is tightly knit. A few of my contemporaries among the local GPs had trained alongside me, many were in a young GP group with me. I have been a doctor to some, and a patient to others. The role of Medical Audit Adviser has given me the opportunity to visit every practice in the area and discuss problems and progress with them. Some recruited and trained nurses to a high level in the 1980s. Some practices have borrowed and invested enormous sums of money to create purpose-built surgeries. Some have spent hours summarizing notes and learning to use desktop computers. Each partner in the practice has a different attitude to these changes. When I considered the enormous variety of approaches to delivering primary care, I became keen to learn more about the process of change.

Introduction

The diffusion of innovation is a new topic for general practice. This chapter will address the following questions:

1. What are innovations and how do they proceed?
2. What determines the rate at which innovations spread?
3. What are the characteristics of individuals or groups associated with a willingness to change?
4. Does the adoption of a change follow a predictable pattern?
5. Can the characteristics of those who take up change at each different stage be described?
6. How do researchers' methodologies affect the picture we get of diffusion of innovation?
7. Is innovation necessarily good?

What are innovations and how do they proceed?

The Oxford English dictionary describes the verb 'innovate' as to 'bring in new methods' or 'make changes'. Changes can be of many kinds, for example, technical changes such as the introduction of computers to assist in data management in general practice. Changes can be practical and behavioural, for example, GPs may decide to use their budgets to employ nurses and transfer to them the skills and the responsibility for health promotion and preventive services.

Technical change may also require behavioural change. GPs who adopt desktop computers may initially feel de-skilled as they attempt to communicate and problem-solve with the patient, whilst simultaneously learning to type and come to terms with a new software system. In the past, the pharmaceutical industry invested one-fifth of its income on promoting doctors' uptake of new drugs, thus attempting to influence their behaviour. Also important are changes in behaviour due to new knowledge, for example, the abandonment of drugs like tetracycline when potential side effects were found to outweigh the benefits. From these examples, it becomes clear that whatever doctors do, or refuse to do, they are taking up a position *vis-à-vis* the changes in knowledge, attitudes and practice which are occurring around them. This is an important process, but a neglected field of research.

Although the study of decision-making in the face of uncertainty is uncommon in medicine, economists have made this a central focus of interest in their own discipline. Their theories evolved around observing and attempting to predict the behaviour of market-makers. In the United States, Von Neumann and Morgenstern (1953) compared decision-makers in the market to gamblers. From a position of uncertainty, market-makers assessed a number of alternatives and weighed up the probability of different outcomes. Rogers (1983) and a group of social scientists later described how changes in agricultural methods and technology spread from research centres in America to farms across the country. Having developed models and made observations, these researchers turned their attention to other sectors of the economy, like health care.

When one considers the change that has taken place in general practice, it becomes clear that innovation is not a one-stage process. Rogers described five possible stages.

Gaining knowledge

First, individuals must obtain knowledge about the possibilities of some new technology or practice. In general practice, this may be achieved by reading the *British Medical Journal*, or the *British Journal of General Practice*, or perhaps more often by reading a summary in the free medical press. Information can also be acquired by attending postgraduate medical centres and conferences, by reading the lay press, and by listening to patients. The availability and access which GPs have to information is important. Stross and Harlan (1979) and Dunn (1981) analyzed to what extent doctors' behaviour had been changed by a definitive clinical trial which demonstrated the beneficial effect of photocoagulation in treating diabetic retinopathy. They found that 18 months after a publication which described the new evidence, practitioners were comparatively unaware of a benefit which they could have been passing on to their patients. Part of the problem seemed to be that the original report was in a comparatively obscure journal which was read mainly by ophthalmologists. It was not until this information was taken up and cited in mainstream journals that physicians and general practitioners began to hear of it. Pharmaceutical-sponsored magazines do attempt to fill this knowledge gap for GPs, but this in itself does not change doctors' behaviour; it is only the first step in the process of change.

Persuasion

The second stage is one of persuasion. Greer (1988) analyzed the diffusion of innovation among doctors by interviewing a large sample of practitioners in both the United States and in Britain. She found that practitioners were sceptical about research. They justified this scepticism in two ways. Firstly, they said that they distrusted academics and scientists, as research was like motherhood, and to the mother there was no such thing as an ugly baby. Secondly, they said that reports of research was often insufficient, and they had no way of knowing whether the patients described in some studies were similar to their own. For this reason, practitioners were more inclined to depend on local social contacts in evaluating novel approaches. An example of this might be the use of nurses in doing cervical smears. When I trained in Canada in the early 1970s, I had seen nurses working as practitioners in family practice. In Britain, Fullard et al. (1987) and Stilwell et al. (1987) wrote papers advocating the use of nurses in ill-health prevention and health promotion tasks, and reported high levels of patient satisfaction with the service. Many practitioners were aware of this at a conceptual level, but in our own district it was not until the late 1980s and early 1990s that most practices began changing the skill mix in their own teams.

Decision-making

Persuasion does not necessarily lead to decision-making, especially in a group practice where some partners may favour a change, while others, for equally cogent reasons, oppose it. An example of this is the investment of resources where benefits accrue only over a long period of time. Creating purpose-built premises and buying computers are major decisions for practices. Older partners may well see themselves being asked to invest their income when there is little hope of return for them, and considerable inconvenience involved in adapting to change. Corporate decision-making of this kind is difficult and may lead to dissolution of partnerships. Polarization may occur between practices, groups with predominantly younger partners becoming increasingly different from those dominated by older partners. In the case of computers, it was not until everyone in the research club I attend had adopted computers, and were using the same hard and software systems, that I was persuaded to adopt computerization.

Implementation

Once a decision has been made to change, it needs to be implemented. This is by no means straightforward. Even if the partners agree, for example, to pay for and choose a desktop computer system, a visit to the practice is likely to show a great deal of variation in its use. Older partners may have it on the desk but not use it, some partners may use it for prescribing only, some use it after the patient has left the room, and others may tap into it with the patient sitting beside them. Even if all the partners are entering information, it is likely that the codes they use will vary, as well as the diagnostic categories. This may make the aggregation of data a hotchpotch, although some practices have achieved accurate recordings for some diseases (Nazareth et al., 1993).

Commitment

After an innovation has been implemented, its continued use may not be confirmed for some time. Perhaps our practice signalled our continuing commitment to computers when we decided to abandon double-entering information on the computer and on the Lloyd George record cards. In contrast, a neighbouring small practice similar to my own introduced computers at the time when they were freely available to data providers, but when the companies required GPs to buy the hardware themselves they gave up the computer, as they perceived insufficient benefits from using it.

What determines the rate at which innovations spread?

Rogers (1983) described five features of an innovation which affect the rate at which it is adopted elsewhere.

Relative advantage

The first feature is the relative advantage which change confers on potential adopters. For example, before changes in government policies in the 1980s and early 1990s the relative advantage of having a practice nurse was insufficient to motivate many GPs to employ them. Then payment for cervical screening stopped being on an item-for-service basis and became dependent on percentage targets met, and practices were rewarded for providing clinics for ill-health prevention and health promotion. The economic incentive in turn increased the relative advantage of having a nurse. In 2 years, the number of whole time equivalent practice nurses doubled (Audit Commission, 1992). This is a demonstration of a change in central policy producing a relative advantage which in turn accelerated the rate of adoption of nurses throughout general practice.

In contrast to this, the role of highly trained nurses in primary care was developed particularly for rural areas of North America, but in urban areas the innovation was not taken up. At McMaster University, Spitzer *et al.* (1974) trained nurses to work alongside and function potentially as an alternative to family practitioners. They demonstrated that families randomly allocated to nurses or doctors had no different outcome in terms of health or satisfaction over 1 year. However, there was no mechanism by which doctors could be spread evenly across the country, and most doctors chose to cluster in metropolitan areas where they competed for patients and were remunerated on an item-for-service basis. In this context, employing nurse practitioners in urban areas had few advantages. Spitzer's study showed that doctors suffered a financial disadvantage if they paid nurses without being reimbursed for their work. Consequently, except in rural areas, the rate of adoption of this innovation has been slow.

Compatibility with current ideas

The second characteristic of an innovation which affects its rate of adoption is its compatibility with current ideas. An example of this is the adoption of large co-operative rotas by GPs in order to meet patients' needs for primary care, not just in the 40 hours worked by most people, but in the additional 128 hours each week. Prior to the inception of the National Health Service in 1946, and the new Charter in 1966, doctors in general practice tended to work in isolation from their colleagues, and they were even more isolated from information about the working patterns of their counterparts abroad. There was a tradition in Britain of doctors having responsibility for patients in general practice 24 hours per day, 365 days per year, which became enshrined in the NHS contract.

By and large, GPs seemed to accept a model which expected them to be on call both day and night until they retired or died. This work ethos developed within the context that most GPs were men, and most had wives who accepted the role of answering the telephone and the door, transmitting messages, and generally supporting their husband and his practice. There were some signs of dysfunction such as an excess of alcohol-related deaths and suicide among doctors, but in the first 30 years of the NHS there seemed to be little reason to change.

In the 1980s and 1990s new strategies became possible, which were more compatible with current ideas. The 1966 Charter had encouraged GPs to work with other GPs and develop teams of nurses, receptionists and so on. The idea of working co-operatively in larger groups gained momentum, and an additional push was provided by the terms of the 1990 contract which allowed larger practices or groups of practices to purchase their own secondary care.

A second strand which changed existing ideas lay in the social context for out-of-hours work and the increasing recruitment of women both as medical students and as young GPs. The 50 per cent or more of young GPs who were women were also spending a significant amount of time doing other work like shopping, cooking and, if they had children, caring for them. In this context, the whole concept of a GP working for patients around the clock, and supported by a wife who was equally devoted to his work became incompatible with existing realities.

Despite this, the change in current ideas which would necessarily precede a change in strategy were slow. Many GPs reported dissatisfaction as they tried to negotiate different time commitment and profit sharing in partnerships (Osler, 1991; Allen, 1992), and studies reported increasing acknowledgement of stress as a result of night calls and the interruption of family life by telephone calls (Sutherland and Cooper, 1992). Perhaps the last straw was growing consumerism and numbers of complaints, which spurred doctors in the 1990s to adopt a group strategy towards meeting patients' needs during night hours and at the weekend. Large co-operatives began taking off and seemed for many reasons more compatible with current ideas. In comparison to some western countries, this innovation was slow to come.

Complexity

The third characteristic which affects the rate of adoption of an innovation is its complexity. A drug representative may teach about the possible advantages of a new therapy, and it is comparatively simple for a GP to adopt the change in his or her prescribing habits. However, the decision to purchase computers, choose one type from amongst rival products, train staff to implement the process, and for GPs to learn to communicate, make decisions and record information during the consultation all involve complex processes. From start to finish, it could take a practice over 5 years to implement such charges.

Suitability for trial

The characteristic of complexity influences the fourth factor affecting the rate of adoption, its trialability. Most of the time, practitioners prefer to see colleagues try out an innovation, and then try it out themselves without too much cost and time loss. In the case of computers, there is a long time delay before GPs can observe their colleagues reaping any benefits and therefore become persuaded to try using computing systems themselves. It is expensive in terms of both time and money for a practice to purchase and develop the use of one computer, together with its software systems, and then either to revert back to traditional methods or convert to a different system.

The problem of objectively assessing the advantages and disadvantages of an innovation is discussed in subsequent chapters. The characteristic of trialability could be applied to the prescription of new drugs. In the 1980s, some drugs like Halcion and Opren seemed to work well in the one-to-one doctor–patient therapeutic transaction. This, together with effective marketing, led to rapid rates of adoption. However, adverse effects were reported in the long term in larger populations, and this led to subsequent discontinuation.

Observability

Rogers described the fifth characteristic affecting the rate of adoption as its observability. Perhaps this feature is the most problematic for GPs. In order to keep in contact and observe what fellow professionals are doing, doctors working in the community are dependent on their own social skills. So the characteristics of the innovation and of the individuals who observe them are to a certain extent linked. GPs will observe that colleagues are managing screening programmes more easily with the help of computer systems if they have colleagues who have computer systems *and* if they socialize with them. Clearly, there is in this process the potential for the creation of a charmed circle of privilege on the one hand, and on the other a vicious circle of isolation and delay in adopting changes which might be advantageous to the practice.

What are the characteristics of individuals or groups associated with a willingness to change?

Bosanquet and Leese (1988) surveyed practitioners in seven different areas in England in order to identify by questionnaire the characteristics of practitioners and practices associated with innovation. They divided the practices into three distinct groups. The markers that they chose of innovativeness in the 1980s were:
1. employing practice nurses,
2. participating in the cost rent scheme and
3. participating in the vocational training scheme.

They designated as innovative those practices which had two of these three characteristics. Where none of the three characteristics were present, the practice was designated as traditional. The remaining practices were designated as intermediate. The investigators were then able to relate the innovativeness of practices to the social characteristics of the partners and the area.

They found that traditional practices were much more likely to be found in less affluent areas and were more likely to be urban. Innovative practices were more frequently found in rural and affluent suburban areas. Innovation was also related to the size of the practice. Large practices of four or more partners were more likely to be innovative than practices with fewer partners. Smaller partnerships were more likely to be traditional. In this context, it is worth knowing that the survey did not include GPs working alone.

Innovation was more common in partnerships with younger doctors. This was particularly noticeable in London. The researchers found that innovative practices were more likely to consist of doctors of British origin, with fewer being of Asian origin. Innovative practices were more likely to consist of doctors with further professional qualifications, particularly membership of the Royal College of General Practitioners. Overall, innovative practices earned more than traditional practices, but the incomes varied a great deal. Doctors working in the Thames Valley and eastern rural areas, earned on average significantly more than doctors working in London and the Midlands, regardless of whether they were innovative or traditional.

The results of this study are consistent with the results of studies of doctors in North America. There is a consistent association between more affluent areas and more highly educated practitioners, who are exposed to new ideas both by travelling to conferences and by local social participation. Doctors in larger scale units are likely to be more able to invest in changes that may be too expensive for smaller scale units to adopt. Bosanquet and Leese's (1988) study was a static cross-sectional one, but it enables us to start making hypotheses about cause and effect.

Does the adoption of a change follow a predictable pattern?

Rogers proposed that the process of adoption of change tended to conform to an S-shaped curve which is illustrated in Figure 11.1.

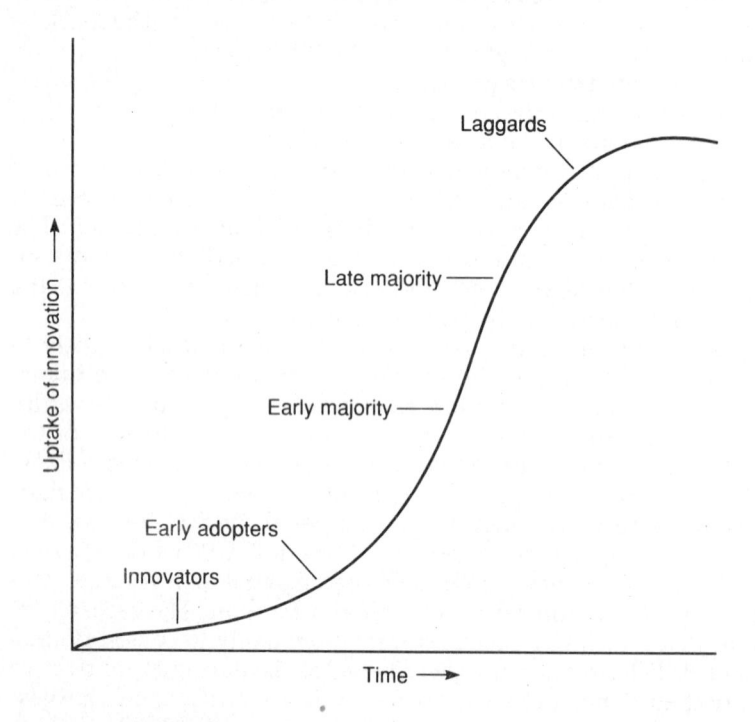

Fig. 11.1 Diffusion of innovation. (From Stocking, 1991. By permission of the King's Fund Centre.)

He suggested that in the beginning the curve – which reflects the rate of uptake – would be relatively flat, as only a few practitioners tried the innovation. The curve might then take off in a more vertical way, as the novelty caught on with the majority of doctors. Finally, the curve would flatten off again, as most doctors had adopted the change. The remaining few practitioners picked up on the change extremely slowly, or not at all. The curve has some implications for answering the question: what types of individuals are involved at the flat early stage of adoption, or at the rapid up phase, or at the flattening off at the top?

Can the characteristics of those who take up change at each different stage be described?

Researchers have concerned themselves with the characteristics of adopters, partly through a wish to describe change, and partly through a desire to promote change in future. Rogers (1983) suggested that highly innovative people can cope with a high degree of uncertainty and are likely to be highly educated. They attend conferences and socialize professionally to a greater degree than others. However, these differences may cause them to be regarded as slightly deviant, and their ideas may be given low credibility by their colleagues.

A second sub-type identified by Rogers were 'idea champions'. These individuals are not necessarily inventors of change, but they have energy and communicating ability. They may canvass in their own area an idea developed somewhere else. In America, Coleman and colleagues (1957) traced the uptake of a new drug by interviewing doctors in four towns. They asked doctors the following questions: to whom did they most often turn for advice? Who were their friends among their colleagues? Who did they generally see most often? The investigators independently analyzed the prescription records of local pharmacies. They found that doctors who were named more often as 'friends' by other doctors used the new drug earlier. There was also a linked relationship between doctors, so that social relationships seemed to exert a 'pull' effect on their uptake of the new drug. The investigators inferred that doctors who were relatively socially isolated and did not have friendships or relationships that encouraged them to adopt change increasingly lagged behind.

Because the general medical community probably regards innovators and idea champions to a certain extent as being *parti pris*, the uptake of change by these two types of individuals will not necessarily lead to the majority changing their behaviour. Becker (1970) postulated that the adoption of change by the majority depended on the behaviour of 'opinion leaders'. An opinion leader has no particular axe to grind *vis-à-vis* a particular innovation. He or she was likely to be more educated, more likely to be regarded as a friend and to attend medical meetings, but also more likely to be relatively conservative, presenting what is regarded as a balanced view. The adoption of change by these opinion leaders generally heralded an upswing in the S-shaped curve.

'Laggards' or 'traditionalists' are described by innovation researchers in rather a deprecating way. This will be discussed further in the next two sections which are concerned with research methodologies, and the social context in which this research has been undertaken.

How do researchers' methodologies affect the picture we get of diffusion of innovation?

I believe that both Rogers' (1983) pioneering work and, in Britain, the work of Bosanquet and Leese (1988) are important both for GPs and for groups like the government who want to influence behaviour. The importance of Bosanquet and Leese's work results partly from their introducing this disciplinary framework of innovation research from America to British general practice (Horder *et al.*, 1986). Bosanquet and Leese's study identified indicators of innovativeness in the 1980s, which would undoubtedly now be different in the 1990s. Having done this, the investigators were able to demonstrate the characteristics of GPs *vis-à-vis* the particular innovations they chose. They also demonstrated that economic rewards are variable, so that innovative practices in London might earn less than traditional practices in the Thames Valley. These findings have important social and political implications.

A limitation of survey research lies in its being a static approach. An alternative research method is that adopted by Greer (1988) and Coleman *et al.* (1957), who interviewed doctors in different places and with regard to particular changes, like the introduction of a new drug. They found that doctors' interpersonal relations and social networks with other doctors were important in determining the rate at which they took up an innovation. These qualitative approaches complement the quantitative approach of Bosanquet and Leese.

In the future, a combined approach might be possible, so that a comparative static or longitudinal view could be obtained. For example, it seems likely that British male graduates have social networks which offer greater opportunities for them to move to high earning large practices in the Thames Valley and eastern rural areas. From a position of comparative advantage, they join groups which are large and who consistently innovate, whatever criteria are applied. These practices, whether they are fundholders or not, are high earners and on the whole provide high quality services to their more middle class clientele. But here is the rub. In inner-city London or the Midlands, patients are more likely to be disadvantaged economically, socially, physically and psychologically and so are in greater need of medical care. But British graduates choose to practise in these communities less often and, even when they do and innovate, they earn less.

In previous chapters, issues of social justice were raised. It is clear that when constructing a system of incentives, medical care cannot be regarded as just another market product. For many reasons, poor communities are unattractive to service providers. But there should be no economic disincentives to practising in these areas.

This leads on to the final subsection:

Is innovation necessarily good?

Rogers (1983) acknowledged that the orientation of researchers towards the diffusion of innovation has from the beginning been biased. The thrust of the research initially was to promote change and the uptake of new agricultural technology and practices, from research centres to the periphery. Subsequently, this 'innovation is good' perspective was perpetuated by American public agencies studying the introduction of medical technologies like contraception to developing countries. Change, and those who promoted it, were construed as the 'goodies', whilst those who resisted it were described using all sorts of pejorative terms. Subsequently, the researchers themselves realized that this was naïve.

Many changes in medicine, which were perceived to be progressive at the time, have subsequently been abandoned or even attacked as harmful to health. Physicians rightly hold variable attitudes towards the introduction of new drugs, or to screening for well patients. Often, change has occurred before there was adequate evidence to support it, almost like a fashion in new clothes. Change does not necessarily equate with progress, and even if it did an equitable distribution of medical care will not result from criticizing the traditionalists.

Finally, it seems to me that when one considers each change in practice, it is likely that the character types described by researchers may not be constant. Practitioners may adopt different attitudes in different spheres. For example, in my own district, I probably acted as an idea champion as far as the introduction of nurses was concerned. My colleagues led the way when it came to expensive innovations like computers, whereas I may have functioned as an opinion leader or may have been just one of the many who adopted computers on the upswing of the S-shaped curve. When it comes to introducing new drugs, I am probably a laggard. This variable behaviour towards innovations would require sophisticated theories and strategies in order to explain and measure what is going on.

Innovations theory has hitherto been developed in a social context, since innovativeness in itself was seen to be politically correct. It is difficult to take a neutral stance and not identify with the assumption that innovation is good. It is even more difficult to tease through the consequences, in terms of medical care for patients, of rewarding innovators and economically punishing those who are not. The issue of the dependence of theory and research on values will be taken up in the final chapter.

References

Allen, I. (1992) *Part-time Working in General Practice*. London: Policy Studies Institute.
Audit Commission (1992) *The Community Revolution*. London: HMSO.
Becker, M. H. (1970) Factors affecting diffusion of innovations among health professionals. *American Journal of Public Health* 60: 294–304.
Bosanquet, N. & Leese, B. (1988) Family doctors and innovation in general practice. *British Medical Journal* 296: 1576–1580.
Coleman, J., Katz, E. & Menzel, H. (1957) The diffusion of an innovation among physicians. *Sociometry* 20: 253–270.
Dunn, D. R. F. (1981) Dissemination of the published results of an important clinical trial: An analysis of the citing literature. *Bulletin Medical Library Association* 69: 301–306.
Fullard, E., Fowler, G. & Gray, M. (1987) Promoting prevention in primary care: Controlled trial of low technology, low cost approach. *British Medical Journal* 294: 1080–1082.
Greer, A. L. (1988) The state of the art versus the state of the science. *International Journal of Technology Assessment in Health Care* 4: 5–26.
Horder, J., Bosanquet, N. & Stocking, B. (1986) Ways of influencing the behaviour of general practitioners. *Journal of the Royal College of General Practitioners* 36: 517–521.
Nazareth, I., King, M., Haines, A., Rangel, L. & Myers, S. (1993) Accuracy of diagnosis of psychosis on general practice computer systems. *British Medical Journal* 307: 32–34.
Osler, K. (1991) Employment experiences of vocationally trained doctors. *British Medical Journal* 303: 762–764.
Rogers, E. M. (1983) *Diffusion of Innovations*. New York: Free Press.
Spitzer, W. O., Sackett, D. L., Sibley, J. C., Roberts, R. S., Gent, M., Kergin, D. et al. (1974) The Burlington randomized trial of the nurse practitioner. *New England Journal of Medicine* 290: 251–256.
Stilwell, B., Greenfield, S., Drury, M. & Hull, F. M. (1987) A nurse practitioner in general practice: Working style and pattern of consultations. *Journal of the Royal College of General Practitioners* 37: 154–157.
Stocking, B. (1991) Bringing about change. In: Salvage, J. (ed.) *Nurse Practitioners: Working for Change in Primary Health Care Nursing*. London: King's Fund Publishing Office.
Stross, J. K. & Harlan, W. (1979) The dissemination of new medical information. *Journal of the American Medical Association* 241: 2622–2624.
Sutherland, V. J. & Cooper, C. L. (1992) Job stress, satisfaction, and mental health among general practitioners before and after introduction of the new contract. *British Medical Journal* 304: 1545–1548.
Von Neumann, J. & Morgenstern, O. (1953) *Theory of Games and Economic Behaviour*, 3rd edn. New York: Wiley (formerly Princeton: Princeton University Press).

12

Changing the Skill Mix in the Primary Care Team

> At the Medical Audit Advisory Group (MAAG) meeting, we discussed how the primary care team can meet the needs of patients and improve care for patients whom, we are told, should get a 'seamless' service.

Introduction

GPs are constantly being told about areas of need that have been hitherto relatively neglected, like monitoring patients with epilepsy, and they have already increased the range of services they provide for patients with, for example, hypertension, diabetes and asthma. These services were formally provided by doctors in training under consultant supervision in out-patient departments and are now provided in primary care. This shift of functions across the interface has on the whole been welcomed by patients as it provides more continuity of care, and it has been welcomed by the medical professional provided that similar standards of care can be provided in general practice.

If shifts in care provision are to continue from tertiary to secondary to primary care, general practitioners will need to rethink their own position *vis-à-vis* skill mix, and negotiate with other members of the primary care team in order to allocate tasks appropriately. In the past, this has been done on rather an intuitive basis and practices have varied considerably. In the future, practice teams will need to be more clear about what they mean by skill mix, need, medical care and medical outcomes, cost and relative benefits of particular activities, and what evidence there is about the activities and potential roles of various members of the practice team.

Skill mix

Bevan *et al.* (1991) described skill mix as being 'about identifying the range of tasks and responsibilities involved in providing care within a particular speciality, what levels are involved and therefore who is appropriate to carry them out.' Skill mix goes beyond looking at grades within one professional group to look at 'the mix of different professions and other staff types appropriate to provide the required service,... thus it means considering where the roles of different grades within one staff group meet the boundaries of the roles of other staff groups. A skill mix review is not just about the relationship between qualified staff and unqualified social workers – it is also about the borders between, for example, what doctors and midwives do; or the borders between what nurses, health visitors' and other workers do (Bevan *et al.*, 1991). Bevan *et al.* proposed a client-centred approach in which providers first defined what services their population required. The providers could then determine what tasks needed to be done in order to perform this work well and economically and achieve specified outcomes. The providers could then go on to look at the general and specific skills and competencies needed to perform to that level, formulate job descriptions, and decide on training and selection procedures and assessment.

Need

This approach might be easier to follow when a new service is provided. It would be extremely difficult to adopt this approach where many professional groups have been working relatively autonomously in primary care and have to a certain extent carved up the territory. However, starting with this approach does make it clear that GPs need to know the strengths and weaknesses of other concepts like 'need'. Need is a word frequently used about patients. One might assume therefore that it had an agreed definition. Wise doctors acknowledge that where there are many different treatments for one condition, there is probably little convincing evidence of the efficacy of any of them. They may experience a certain sinking feeling on learning that social administrators have been defining and debating the concept of need for over 30 years. Culyer and Wagstaff (1992) state,

> 'it is hard to see why someone who is sick can sensibly be said to need health care regardless of the latter's ability to improve the person's health ... the concept of need is inherently consequentialist or instrumental; an entity can be said to be needed only insofar as it is a necessary condition and there is some ultimate goal to be obtained. An alternative, but equivalent way of stating this necessary condition for a need to exist

is that there should be an expected capacity to benefit from the consumption of resources.'

Defining the needs of patients raises questions about the outcome of interventions. Measuring need raises further problems. Wilkin and his colleagues (1992) stated that,

> 'measures of need are . . . not neutral objective descriptions of people. They incorporate value-judgements about what should be accepted as appropriate goals, and what constitutes deficiency from these goals.'

Implicit judgements, they said, are rarely made explicit. They concern a) the standard against which deficiency or need is to be assessed, and b) who should decide what constitutes a need. So far as the standards are concerned, at least three options are available:
1. each can be assessed against some ideal,
2. each can be defined in terms of some minimum, or
3. they can be assessed by reference to a comparison with standards that are achieved in other areas.

The question of who should decide what constitutes a need raises a further problem. On the one hand, consumers may decide what they feel to be their needs and their expectations will vary enormously (Ong, 1991). Older people in the lower socio-economic groups generally have lower expectations of health status and health care (Cartwright and Anderson, 1981). But many people would agree that according to the principle of justice they should not necessarily get less care on this account. Secondly, professionals can define patients' needs. In the past, the provision of medical care has tended to be supply led; need was defined in terms of what professionals had to offer. Thirdly, society or representatives of society can be asked to assess needs using procedures like the quality adjusted life years (QALYS) (Fitzpatrick *et al.*, 1992) or saved young life equivalent procedures (SAVE) (Nord, 1992).

From this discussion, it is clear that need is not a transparent term. There is no single agreed criterion by which it can be assessed. Despite this lack of consensus, the concept of need may link medical care with health status. The economist Evans (1984) stated that it is generally accepted that for most people, most of the time, health status is primarily dependent on sanitation, diet and shelter – the complex effect summarized as 'lifestyle and environment'. He pointed out that it is health as a status rather than health care, as a commodity, which is of value to its users.

> 'The direct effects of most if not all health services on their user's well-being, independent of their anticipated health effects, is negative. Dentistry, drugs, diagnostic and therapeutic interventions, hospital stays, are frequently uncomfortable or frightening in and of themselves. Few, indeed, would choose to propose them in the absence of expected health benefit.'

Recognition of the mediating role of medical care enables us to recognize the possibility of over and under-utilization. Use of the types of care which an informed provider might reasonably expect to do the patient no good, or even harm, represent over-utilization from an economic standpoint. Under-utilization, by contrast, implies that some levels or types of care are not being supplied and used which could increase the health status of some patients enough to justify their cost.

Efficacy and cost

The questions to ask before starting or continuing a medical act or programme are: does it work? Is it effective for the purposes claimed? These are fundamental epidemiological questions which Cochrane (1972) put on the health policy map over 20 years ago. Many services offered in primary care may yield no improvement in anyone's health status, and it may not be worth buying them at any (positive) price.

Enthoven (1980) described a relationship between the collection of activities described as health care or medical services and the resources needed to provide them. He pointed out that the health care industry, or specific sub-components of it, may extend resources well beyond the point at which intervention ceased to be effective, yet each participant may act on imperfect information with the best of intentions and be highly resistant to the suggestion that they are practising 'flat-of-the-curve' medicine. This is illustrated in the diagram in Chapter 9.

Labour costs and numbers

Appraising the skill mix needed by any team therefore ideally requires a consideration of what patients might need. This involves an estimation of how they might benefit from care. As there are many different professional groups working within primary care, the allocation of tasks among them will depend to a certain extent on an appraisal of the skills they have and to a certain extent on the cost of employing them to carry out particular tasks. In Chapter 9, it was pointed out that the average GP worked or was on call for 72 hours a week, and in 1994 the average net remuneration for GPs was £42,000 per annum. In the same year, Heath (1994) pointed out that nurses work an average of 37.5 hours per week, and at the top end of the scale they may earn up to £23,750 per annum. At these rates, and if all hours of work were considered to be of equal value, GPs would be earning on average £11 per hour and nurses at the top end of the scale £12 per hour. Seen in this context, the transfer of work from doctors to nurses working at the top end of the pay scale may not be cost-saving and may need to be considered more in terms of the availability of staff to carry out particular tasks who have the skills required for these particular tasks.

In the early 1990s, there were approximately 26,000 full-time equivalent general practitioners working in England and Wales (Economic Research Unit, 1992). There were approximately 20,000 whole time equivalent personnel working in the district nursing service, 52 per cent of whom were qualified sisters (Lightfoot et al., 1992). There were approximately 12,000 whole time equivalents working in the health visitors service, 87 per cent of whom were qualified sisters. And approximately 10,000 equivalent whole time practice nurses were employed directly by general practitioners (Audit Commission, 1992). Small groups of nurse specialists working in the community included midwives and nurses working in psychiatry, psychogeriatrics, MacMillan teams, schools, family planning clinics and on drug abuse programmes. When the numbers in nursing and medical groups are added up, the ratio of nurses to doctors working in the community was probably about 2 to 1.

Practice nurses

When tasks and responsibilities are being distributed in primary care, an important but difficult challenge is to assess the third general area described by Bevan et al. (1991), which involves examining the potential for change in the context of the training and assessment provided for the professional groups involved. Ross and Bower (1992) and Ross et al. (1994) examined the work of practice nurses in the South-West Thames region. They found that the average practice nurse was in her 40s and worked approximately half time. Half of the nurses had worked as practice nurses for less than 2 years, and half were employed on the G grade. Practice nurses were often the first point of contact with the public. The majority of the respondents gave clinical advice over the telephone (92 per cent), dealt with casual attenders (84 per cent) and were the first contact in emergencies (71 per cent). Nearly one-half of the practice nurses fulfilled criteria for defining them as independent practitioners, in that they prescribed within an agreed protocol or made home visits for initial assessments.

Ross and Bower (1992) were interested to know the extent to which nurses had been formally trained and assessed in the provision of care over a range of tasks and responsibilities. They found that 62 per cent of the nurses who were providing family planning advice held an appropriate qualification. Twelve per cent of nurses providing asthma care had an appropriate formal training or English National Board Certificate, and only 1 per cent of the nurses providing diabetic care had completed a formally recognized course. On the other hand, one-quarter of the nurses were qualified as midwives, but they did not provide antenatal and postnatal care, presumably due to concern that they might be taking over tasks currently undertaken by midwives, or to a perceived inability to keep up to date in the subject.

Ross and Bower (1992) also asked the nurses how they perceived their roles as changing in the future. They found that 85 per cent of nurses reported that they were thinking about developing or expanding their role. The tasks and responsibilities that practice nurses wanted to take on were: counselling skills, health promotion, clinical nursing roles, treatment protocols, information technology, interviewing skills and research.

Cross-sectional studies such as this one are important in evaluating the skill mix of this professional group. The evidence suggests that the workforce and responsibilities of practice nurses have been changing rapidly. Practice nurses seem to have demonstrated unusual degrees of flexibility and willingness to take on tasks which were previously not performed, or which were performed by other members of the primary health care team. An important concern is whether they have sufficient training and assessment systems to perform this work well.

Primary care services

From the point of view of the general practitioner, there are many services which the primary care team need to offer. These include: responding to patients' demands for care for acute problems seen at the surgery and seen in their homes during normal office hours, during the night and at weekends. Secondly, there are preventive and health education responsibilities like providing family planning advice, cervical screening and immunization services. Thirdly, there is a whole expanding area of monitoring chronic problems such as hypertension, diabetes, asthma and epilepsy.

Acute needs and services

The services which are provided either outside the general practice in patient's homes, or outside normal office hours, represent a particular logistic challenge for general practitioners. Evidence about this has often been derived from general practitioners measuring what they do in their own particular practices. Whewell and colleagues (1983) studied the changing patterns of home visiting during office hours in one practice. Between 1969 and 1980, they found that home visits had decreased by 41 per cent over the period and that there had also been a 31 per cent decrease in requests from patients. The greatest decrease in home visits requested during the day was for those aged less than 1 year old, the greatest increase was for those aged over 65 years.

Marsh and his colleagues (1987) measured the content of night and weekend work provided by the same practice. They found that 59 per cent of calls were managed by telephone, 37 per cent by home visits and 5 per cent by out-of-hours surgery attendance. When they looked at the age distribution of out-of-hours calls, they found that the practice was five times as likely to receive calls about patients between 0 and 4 years old, and twice as likely to receive calls about patients over 80 years of age.

The investigators analyzed the nature of the problems which were presented to doctors at night and during the weekend. They found that 16 per cent of patients had a problem for which they were already receiving treatment, and 70 per cent of these calls were managed by telephone. Eighteen per cent of incoming calls were about upper respiratory tract infections, and 70 per cent of these were managed by telephone. Twelve per cent of calls were about acute gastro-intestinal upsets, and 70 per cent of these were managed by telephone. When the investigators looked at what kind of treatment was given, they found that 11 per cent of patients required simple analgesics, and 80 per cent of these were managed by telephone. Eleven per cent required gastric management, and 70 per cent of these were managed by telephone.

The picture emerging from this evidence reflects changing social, economic and demographic trends. Young, geographically mobile mothers are likely to live further from their own mothers and extended support network, and they are more likely to call on the GP for advice about young children at night and at weekends. These people are increasingly likely to have access to transport and are able to bring their child to the surgery. On the other hand, there is a need expressed increasingly by elderly and immobile patients for home visits. Much of this need is for good advice and the support that might be given by a well trained nurse or by a doctor.

Nurse practitioners

In the context of the assessment and management of acute and subacute problems, it may be worth considering transferring tasks and responsibilities from doctors to nurse practitioners. The model of a nurse practitioner as an alternative gate-keeper or triager has been developed to a greater extent in North America for two reasons. There is no legislation to compel doctors to distribute themselves evenly in Canada or the United States, and many rural communities are therefore without a doctor. Secondly, the role of physician's assistant has been developed in the military services. After being demobilized from the services, these people have looked for work with greater scope for decision-making; work which is autonomous and independent from medical practitioners.

How can a distribution of skills and tasks among nurse practitioners be evaluated? This question was posed through a social experiment described in Chapter 11 (Spitzer et al., 1974). Two experienced practice nurses both underwent training to learn how to evaluate patients' presenting problems and how to choose treatment options. The experiment was undertaken over an 18-month period in two practices. In the pre-trial period, measurements were made of patients' physical function, daily activities and disability using standardized questionnaires. Families were then randomized on a two-to-one ratio to doctors or nurses. Very few patients refused to accept their allocation. During the year in which the experiment was undertaken a time and motion study was undertaken in each practice, and ten indicator 'tracer' conditions were used to assess management and drugs prescribed.

When an analysis was undertaken of the ten indicator conditions, no significant difference was found between the general practitioners and nurse practitioners in terms of management and prescriptions. Two-thirds of nurse practitioners visits were made without the need to consult general practitioners. When the study was completed, no significant difference was found in physical function, daily activities and disability between patients assigned to the general practitioners and patients assigned to the nurses. The investigators concluded that 'the results demonstrate the nurse practitioner can provide first contact primary clinical care as safely and effectively, with as much satisfaction to patients, as the family practitioner.'

Similar training to that provided for nurse practitioners at McMaster University is provided in the United Kingdom by the Royal College of Nursing (1990). The training is offered to experienced nurses and includes taking case histories, physical examination and pharmacy. Recruits come from the various nurse sub-specialists working within the community, including practice nurses, district nurses and health visitors.

As the number of practice nurses has doubled, the clinical role of health visitors has been eroded. Practices have taken on the tasks of immunization and vaccination, and providing disease prevention and health education advice to young mothers. In this last area, the role of health visitors has come increasingly under threat as district and GP budget holders ask themselves what they, as purchasers, are going to get in return for their financial outlay? But young mothers do still feel they need advice and support, and general practitioners may not have the most appropriate skills and the time to provide this. One-quarter of new consultations with general practitioners are for respiratory infections, and a large proportion of their work is concerned with minor illnesses like coughs and colds in children. Much of this service provision may conform to what Enthoven (1980) described as 'flat of the curve medicine'. There is little evidence that doctors benefit patients by seeing them with self-remitting symptoms, and many patients do not consult for similar complaints (Morrell and Wale, 1976). In this context, there may be an argument for including the health visitor in the primary health care team through a change in training and a modified role. Health visitors already have expertise in advising mothers about normal childhood problems. They could become nurse practitioners for the under 5s in the short and medium term, whilst retaining an opportunistic and systematic role with regard to disease prevention and health promotion for the same patient population. Such a shift in tasks and responsibilities would require evaluation, but the evidence from Canada (Spitzer et al., 1974) suggests there would be little change in outcomes or patient satisfaction.

Prevention and health education

When considering the preventive and health promotion role of general practice, health visitors could have a role which is more integrated in the primary care team. Ross and Bower (1992) and Ross et al. (1994) found that practice nurses are perceived to lack the training for their preventive and health promotion role. In 1994, the Imperial Cancer Research Fund OXCHECK Study Group showed that systematic health checks by practice nurses had little positive effect in terms of reducing risk factors for cardiovascular disease. The Family Heart Study Group (1994) also systematically tested the role of nurses. They adopted a central training programme for the nurses in client-centred counselling about lifestyle within families. These nurses functioned as teachers in a similar way to health visitors. This programme led to a small reduction in risk factors for coronary events, which the group pointed out were associated with more intense resource input in terms of training and time for the nurses. It is not clear whether primary prevention of vascular disease can ever be cost-effective. It may be that patients will resist systematic attempts to change their lifestyles. It may, however, be the case that more could be achieved if health visitors were drawn into the practice team, where they could teach practice nurses the communication skills that may be more effective in promoting adult learning and behaviour change. This whole area needs more research.

Managing chronic conditions

The third major area in which the primary care team has tasks and responsibilities is in managing chronic conditions, such as hypertension, asthma, diabetes and epilepsy. As general practitioners have taken on the responsibility for pro-active and systematic monitoring of these patients, the task of seeing them has tended to be delegated to practice nurses using protocols. However, it is not clear from studies like those undertaken by Ross and Bower (1992) and Ross *et al.* (1994) that practice nurses have been adequately trained and assessed to fulfil these roles. There is still a considerable range in the personnel considered suitable for monitoring these patients from practice nurses, to general practitioners, to specialists. It is not clear which professional groups or which combination of personnel are best equipped to manage these conditions. On the one hand, doctors may have greater knowledge and skills, and they may wish to continue to be primary carers for these patient groups. On the other hand, Tuckett *et al.* (1985) have shown that GPs rather infrequently share their expert knowledge with their patients or provide the reactive explanations that these people need in order to manage their conditions themselves. Runyon (1975) found that nurses specially trained to educate and counsel patients with chronic problems like hypertension and diabetes achieved improved outcomes in terms of blood glucose, blood pressure levels and prevention of hospitalization.

As the care of these patients with chronic disease is increasingly shifted across the interface from hospital care to general practice, it is important that workers in primary care identify the appropriate combination of expert knowledge and communication skills and time, and how they might be provided to meet the needs of these patient groups. On the one hand, doctors might decide that providing time for their patients was a priority and that they needed to improve their skills in providing client-centred counselling. On the other hand, nurses might be provided with more training about particular conditions, or teams with different skills might work together in a systematic and integrated way such as that described by Kopersky (1992) for patients with diabetes. In the mid-1990s, a shift in care for these patients has been achieved, but the style and quality with which this care is delivered must be extremely variable. Since there is variation, observation and evaluation are needed to assess the strengths and weaknesses of different models.

District nurses

Thinking on and evaluation of teamwork occur at particular points in time. It is difficult in this context to take account of the longer term implications of shifts in tasks and responsibilities in terms of training and assessment.

Lightfoot *et al.* (1992) found that district nurses were able to define their role precisely and identify tasks which could be delegated to less skilled personnel. This is reflected in the high ratio of less skilled to more skilled workers in the district nursing service. The expanding need for clinical nursing in the community has to a certain extent required this flexibility in approach to delegation. The need for clinical nursing in the community is likely to increase in the next decade, with changes in demographic trends and redistribution of work from secondary to primary care. It is expected that there will be a 33 per cent increase in the over-85s. Day care surgery and early discharge policies will be increasingly implemented, and there will be more demand for terminal care services to be provided in the community. Some fundholding groups of practitioners are now purchasing the skills of district nurses directly. As part of this integrative process, district and practice nurses will be able to decide how to perform the clinical tasks for which they are responsible. Hitherto, the continuation of traditional working patterns has meant that district nurses still see patients in their homes, even when they were sufficiently mobile to come to the surgery. The Value for Money Study Team (1992) found that one-quarter of nurses' time was spent travelling. When district and practice nurses are managing together, it will be possible for them to divide up the work rather as GPs do, with some seeing patients in the surgery and some making home visits, depending on the patients' needs and their mobility.

The Value for Money Study Team (1992) measured how district nurses spent their time. They questioned the way time was allocated to management, training of juniors, clinical practice and other work. The question of how much time senior practitioners need to spend on management and training, and how much time they need to spend on clinical practice in order to sustain their own skills, has no clear answers. A study by Carr-Hill *et al.* (1992) of nurses working in hospitals suggested that a mix with lower grades and skills was associated with lower quality of care. These concerns about quality of care and skills need to be addressed in primary care also.

Lightfoot and colleagues' (1992) report on community nursing described an approach to the setting of objectives which depended on a resource-led historical tradition. Their report was an indictment of a professional group which they said lacked the facility of self-criticism and failed to ask questions about what they ought to be doing and where they ought to be going. However, this uncritical historical approach to practice has been adopted just as much by general practitioners and hospital doctors as it has by community nurses. Criticism, questioning and measuring are skills which are not widespread. And they are not generally acquired with clinical on-the-job training. The model of apprenticeship is a popular and apparently cost-effective approach to acquiring knowledge, skills and attitudes, and this model of learning has been used for training nurses, doctors and teachers. But it has disadvantages in that it may encourage an historical or functionalist view among learners. This teaching style implicitly says: what was good enough for the trainer is good enough for the trainee. In general practice, the need for the trainee to get a trainer's report and certificate of competence may discourage new recruits from rocking the boat with new ideas.

When Kuhn (1970) analyzed the process of change, invention and innovation in the scientific world, he suggested that new recruits, and those at the edge of a scientific discipline, are those most able to provide and accept new ideas. He pointed out that fundamental changes take a long time to occur in the scientific world and may even require the older generation to die out. In the medical world, a model of learning which depends on apprenticeship will also tend to discourage criticism, questioning, new ideas and therefore change. Some doctors and nurses who have undergone traditional training in primary care may wish to go on and acquire further skills. Some of these needs can be met in the context of primary care or general practice Master's Degree courses (Ridsdale and Walker, 1990) and other postgraduate programmes (Koppel and Pietroni, 1991).

If questioning, innovation and evaluation are to be fostered in the primary care team, this will require support in terms of time and resources.

References

Audit Commission (1992) *Homeward Bound: A New Course for Community Health*. London: HMSO.
Bevan, S., Stock, J. & Waite, R. K. (1991) *Choosing an Approach to Reprofiling and Skill Mix*. Institute of Manpower Studies.
Carr-Hill, R., Dixon, P., Gibbs, I. et al. (1992) *Skill Mix and the Effectiveness of Nursing Care*. University of York: Centre for Health Economics.
Cartwright, A. & Anderson, R. (1981) *General Practice Revisited*. London: Tavistock Publication.
Cochrane, A. L. (1972) *Effectiveness and Efficiency*. London: Nuffield Provincial Hospitals Trust.
Culyer, A. J. & Wagstaff, A. (1992) *Need, Equity and Equality in Health and Health Care*. York: University of York Centre for Health Economics.
Economic Research Unit (1992) GP manpower in England and Wales. *Quarterly Bulletin of the British Medical Association*, no. 7: 3.
Enthoven, A. C. (1980) *Health Plan*. Reading, Massachusetts. Addison-Wesley Publishing Company.
Evans, R. (1984) *Strained Mercy*. Toronto: Butterworth.

Family Heart Study Group (1994) Randomized controlled trial evaluating cardiovascular screening and intervention in general practice: Principal results of British family heart study. *British Medical Journal* 308: 313–320.

Fitzpatrick, R., Fletcher, A., Gore, S., James, D., Spiegel Halter, D. & Cox, D. (1992) Quality of life measures in health care. *British Medical Journal* 305: 1074–1077.

Heath, I. (1994) Skill mix in primary care. *British Medical Journal* 308: 993–994.

Imperial Cancer Research Fund OXCHECK Study Group (1994) Effectiveness of health checks conducted by nurses in primary care: Results of the OXCHECK study after one year. *British Medical Journal* 308: 308–312.

Kopersky, M. (1992) How effective is systematic care of diabetic patients? A study in one general practice. *British Journal of General Practice* 42: 508–511.

Koppel, J. I. & Pietroni, R. G. (1991) *Higher Professional Courses in the United Kingdom*. Royal College of General Practitioners, Occasional Paper 51.

Kuhn, T. S. (1970) *The Structure of Scientific Revolutions*. Chicago: University of Chicago Press.

Lightfoot, J., Baldwin, S. & Wright, K. (1992) *Community Nursing Study Stage One, Report on a Study of Establishment Setting and Review for District Nursing and Health Visiting Services*. University of York: Social Policy Research Unit.

Marsh, G. N., Hornes, R. A. & Channing, D. M. (1987) A study of telephone advice in managing out-of-hours calls. *Journal of the Royal College of General Practitioners* 37: 301–304.

Morrell, D. C. & Wale, C. J. (1976) Symptoms perceived and recorded by patients. *Journal of the Royal College of General Practitioners* 26: 398–403.

Nord, E. (1992) An alternative to QALY, the saved young life equivalent (SAVE). *British Medical Journal* 305: 875–877.

Ong, B. N. (1991) Researching needs in district nursing. *Journal of Advanced Nursing* 16: 638–647.

Ridsdale, L. & Walker, M. (1990) Continuing medical education at a university – evaluation of an MSc programme in general practice. *Journal of the Royal Society of Medicine* 83: 702–703.

Ross, F. & Bower, P. (1992) *A Study of Practice Nurses Working in South West Thames Regional Health Authority: The Current and Future Activities, Learning and Professional Development Needs of Practice Nurses*. London: Department of General Practice, St George's Hospital Medical School.

Ross, F. M., Bower, P. J. & Sibbald, B. S. (1994) Practice nurses: Characteristics, workload and training needs. *British Journal of General Practice* 44: 15–18.

Royal College of Nursing (1990) *Nurse Practitioners' Diploma in Primary Health Care*.

Runyon, J. W. (1975) The Memphis chronic disease program: Comparisons in outcome and the nurse's extended role. *Journal of the American Medical Association* 231: 264–267.

Spitzer, W. O., Sackett, D. L., Sibley, J. C., Roberts, R. S., Gert, M., Kergin, D. et al. (1974) The Burlington randomized trial of the nurse practitioner. *New England Journal of Medicine*: 251–256.

Tuckett, D., Boulton, M., Olson, C. & Williams, A. (1985) *Meetings Between Experts*. London: Tavistock Publications.

Value for Money Study Team (1992) *The Nursing Skill Mix in the District Nursing Service*. London: HMSO.

Whewell, J., Marsh, G. N. & McNay, R. A. (1983) Changing patterns of home visiting in the North of England. *British Medical Journal* 286: 1259–1961.

Wilkin, D., Hallam, L. & Doggett, M.-A. (1992) *Measures of Need and Outcome for Primary Health Care*. Oxford: Oxford University Press.

13

Critical Appraisal

> In the evening after work, I put my feet up and settled down to some reading. Earlier in the week I had been sent two papers, one by the *British Medical Journal* and one by the *British Journal of General Practice*. They were both on topics that interested me. The editors had asked my opinion about their suitability for publication, and each of them had included checklists of their criteria for eligibility. (See Appendices.)

Why do it?

When doctors finish training in general practice, they still may have 30–40 years of clinical practice ahead of them before retirement. During this time medical knowledge will be changing, and failure to continue to learn will lead to a declining ability to inform patients about what is on offer at the time. For this reason, learning how to assess new evidence as it is described in the literature is a prerequisite to future learning and practice. The General Medical Council now recommends that critical appraisal should be taught at undergraduate level, but some doctors will have missed the boat. A few doctors still feel that critical appraisal is something practised by academics in private. This is no longer the case. Trainees demonstrate skills in critical reading in order to pass the Critical Reading part of the examination to become members of the Royal College of General Practitioners.

The College emblem combines caring with science. Preparing for and passing this exam may help to prevent future GPs having only one (*caritas*) of these two components. Once doctors become immersed in practice, they can neglect their own needs, including that of continuing education, and they may burn out. Mastering the skill of critical appraisal may help prevent this.

The aim of this chapter is to describe some criteria against which research papers can be assessed. Where possible, the examples will be drawn from the papers which have been cited in previous chapters.

How to do it

There is no great mystery surrounding the ability to read critically. It requires some knowledge, but it is above all a skill, and like playing the piano, the more a person practises, the better he or she becomes. It also helps to have seen through a project oneself, and this is something most trainees are now encouraged to do. A hands on approach to data management helps by providing practical experience in simple statistical methods such as choosing between a median and a mean, and insight into how other people manage their data.

One approach when trying to improve one's own skill in reading papers is for readers to imagine that they are being asked to act as a referee for a major journal. Journal editors often ask referees to appraise a paper because they have carried out research on related topics in the past, on the principle: set a thief to catch a thief. For the papers to be published, both the referees and the editor have decided that, compared with other papers that have been submitted, there is something interesting or useful presented in this paper. Critical appraisal is therefore not just about identifying the negative aspects of a study. There are strengths and weaknesses in every paper. The critical reader needs criteria with which to identify and assess these in a balanced way.

Assessment criteria

When learning the skill of critical appraisal, some guidelines and source materials are particularly useful. The *British Medical Journal* and the *British Journal of General Practitioners* both produce checklists for referees, and copies of these are provided in the Appendices. Sackett and colleagues have produced an excellent chapter called 'How to read a clinical journal' in their book on clinical epidemiology (1985). This provides detailed instructions on how to appraise different papers reporting different types of study. Medical practitioners cannot be expected to have sophisticated statistical knowledge, but a checklist can help. A good one is provided in Chapter 10 of Gardner and Altman's book *Statistics with Confidence* (1989).

A structure within a structure – the wrapping

A paper consists of two components. The first is the literary product itself. It has its own structure and clarity or opaqueness of style. A paper secondly provides a description of what investigators think they have found out and how. Bradford Hill (Anon, 1965) described the structure of a paper as answering four questions: why did they start? (Introduction), how did they do it? (Methods), what did they find? (Results), and what does it mean? (Discussion). The first, and a recurring consideration for the critical reader is: to what extent are Bradford Hill's questions answered clearly, and are the answers in the places the reader expects to find them?

1. *Introduction.* Is there a clear description of the problem, a review of the literature, and are the questions or aims stated clearly, usually in the final paragraph?
2. *Methods.* Are they so clearly described that the study could be replicated by someone else?
3. *Results.* Are these clearly expressed?
4. *Discussion.* Is this clear?

Lack of clarity may be due either to researchers hedging or to a lack of fluency in their written English. Those who choose to enter science or medicine may not have written essays for many years, and this may be a handicap when they want to share their interests and findings with others. A problem sometimes encountered when investigators are trying both to make sense of their findings and cope with writing them up is that they have difficulty putting the information in the conventional compartments which Bradford Hill described. Frequently, a description of some of the methods used will appear in the results section, or new results may emerge in the discussion section. This is confusing for readers. When referees or editors believe a paper is worth publishing, they can and do contribute constructively by pointing out to authors the ectopic parts and by suggesting a re-ordering of information which will improve the clarity of the product.

The contents

The next step for the reader is to analyze the contents of the sections in detail. This process is made easier if precise titles and structured abstracts are used (Haynes *et al.*, 1990). The presence of these can be of considerable help to the reader when deciding whether to spend time and energy on reading a paper.

Introduction

The critical reader will need to ask to what extent:

1. are the questions or aims posed in the introduction relevant and important for general practice?

The papers used to provide evidence in this book were chosen for this reason. Clearly, this involves a subjective judgement, but a reasonable case can be made in their defence. For example, otitis media is a common problem presented to GPs. The decision to prescribe or not to prescribe has important therapeutic and financial implications, as most recipients will be children and therefore receiving prescription drugs at the taxpayers' expense. A trial of the efficacy of antibiotics in children such as that undertaken by Burke et al. (1991) cited in Chapter 3 is therefore potentially important.

2. have the questions already been answered adequately elsewhere? Will this study add something, or have the researchers been reinventing the wheel?

When so little research has been done in general practice, it is unlikely that investigators will be reinventing the wheel. However, where the completion of an MD is essential for career progress, as it is in some parts of hospital medicine, the risk of unnecessary replication is greater. In the case of trialling antibiotics for otitis media, the results of a previous trial (Van Buchem et al., 1981) had found antibiotics were no more useful than a placebo. This trial was undertaken in the Netherlands. If the negative findings were replicated in a study in Britain, it is debatable whether doctors here might be more likely to act on the evidence.

3. was the site and population similar enough to general practice in the NHS, so that, assuming the results are valid, the reader can apply the findings to his or her own practice?

The majority of published papers report evidence about patients treated in hospital, but only a small minority of patients are referred there by GPs. Patients are likely to have been referred partly because their characteristics were different from those who were not referred, so that evidence about tests, treatments and outcomes for them is not necessarily applicable to patients managed solely in primary care. Also, referral pathways may be quite different in other countries, such as the United States, where patients see specialists as their first-line doctor and are then sometimes referred from one specialist to another. It is less likely that these studies will be germane to British general practice.

4. Does the literature review provide a clear description of the background against which these researchers posed their question?

Biomedical journals, and these includes the 'big two' for general practitioners, the *British Medical Journal* and the *British Journal of General Practice,* do not give much priority, or space, for authors to review the current literature and contextualize their research questions. Journals in social science, like *Social Science and Medicine,* give more priority and space to these. If an introduction seems too long, sub-editors in biomedical journals may move parts of it to the discussion section. This may wrongly give readers the impression that facts simply emerged and were made sense of subsequently, rather than that the evidence was produced by a particular group of investigators in circumstances influenced by specific historical, social, theoretical and economic considerations.

Readers need to be aware of the difficulties authors face and look out for other papers which may precede or even follow a report, which may help to situate the evidence presented. For example, the study of tradition and innovation in general practice published by Bosanquet and Leese in 1988 was preceded by a literature review in 1986 (Horder *et al.*). A paper by Butler and Calnan on the relation between list size and the use of time was published in the *British Medical Journal* in 1987. It was followed by a more illuminating series of papers in *Social Science and Medicine* in which the social characteristics of GPs were associated with list size and use of time (Calnan, 1988; Calnan and Butler, 1988; Calnan *et al.*, 1992).

Methods

The critical reader needs to ask to what extent the architecture or design of the study is appropriate for best answering the questions posed in the introduction. Some examples of different study classifications are:
1. observational or experimental,
2. retrospective or prospective,
3. longitudinal or cross-sectional.

Study designs

Observational studies – qualitative
In observational studies, researchers collect information about a subject but do not try to influence events. Some aspects of general practice are more closely related to social science. If doctors want to understand more about what patients think, for example, about hypertension or a stigmatized condition like epilepsy, this information may be acquired through interviewing techniques. The interviewer may use all the skills of a good communicator, allow

patients time and site the interview in a place familiar to them, such as their own home. Good examples of qualitative studies are Morgan and Watkins' (1988) study of patients' views of hypertension, and Scambler's (1989) study of patients with epilepsy. Medical journals have been slow to recognize the value of this kind of research and publish it. A description of the scope of qualitative research and ways of appraising it can be found in a book on primary care research by Norton et al. (1991).

Observational studies – quantitative

When comparatively little is known about a subject, a cross-sectional study in which individuals are observed once can establish baseline information. Investigators doing this may form some initial tentative hypotheses. This may involve the social characteristics of the subjects, and their relationship to the outcome which the investigator is interested in. For example, Coulter and Baldwin (1987) were interested in the uptake of cervical screening at a time when the service was not offered in a systematic way. In Oxford, they were able to show that young women in social class 1 and 2 were much more likely to report a smear having been provided than older women in social class 4 and 5. Another useful application of this method was Bosanquet and Leese's (1988) study of the social characteristics of doctors, their incomes and their tendency to innovate. The results of cross-sectional studies such as these provide food for thought for everyone concerned with the delivery of medical care.

If a GP wanted to know about the effect of list size on workload, it would not be feasible or ethical to allocate doctors randomly to practices with different size lists. In this social context, a cross-sectional study such as the one undertaken by Butler and Calnan (1987) is feasible. But it is important to emphasize the limitations of drawing causal inferences from cross-sectional studies of this kind. Associations could easily be due to unforeseen factors, otherwise known as confounding variables. In the example of workload, women doctors and elderly doctors have smaller lists and on average work shorter hours. It cannot be inferred from this that full-time GPs would necessarily reduce their working hours if their list sizes were reduced.

Retrospective studies

In retrospective studies, information can be derived about past events from existing sources of information or by interview. Retrospective studies can be used to identify possible causes of failure to deliver effective medical care. For example, Ellman and

Chamberlain (1984) studied women with invasive cervical cancer in the South-West Thames region and related this to the women's prior cervical screening status. In the majority of cases, 68 out of 100, no screening had been undertaken. This kind of evidence gave little support to those who believed that the most frequent system failures occurred after patients had undertaken a screening test. The majority of women developing invasive cervical cancer had never been included in a screening system.

When retrospective studies include a comparison group, speculations can sometimes be made about the cause of illness. Beale and Nethercott (1985) used registered patients to analyze the relationship between the threat of redundancy and actual redundancy on the consulting rate and on the referral rate of patients in one practice. The strength of the study lay in the 'natural experiment' of a major plant in the town closing down and the investigators' use of all the patients on the practice list who were not employed there as a comparison group. Beale and Nethercott (1986) also used the different age–sex characteristics of patients to tease out possible differential effects of redundancy on men and women of different ages. Their study was also longitudinal in that observations were made at a series of points over a period of time. In this way, they were able to demonstrate that the threat of redundancy 2 years prior to factory closure was associated with increased consulting behaviour by patients and their families.

Prospective studies
In prospective studies, data are collected from the start of the studies onwards. Investigators can rarely afford to monitor their study group all the time, so prospective studies involve a series of measurements or snapshots taken over time. These studies are important for understanding the causes and natural history of disease. They may or may not involve an intervention in the disease process. Brown and his colleagues' work (Brown and Harris, 1978; Brown et al., 1986) illustrates the superiority of a prospective study for teasing out the causes of depression. In their initial study, the investigators measured stresses and supports on one occasion. On the basis of their findings they suggested that when stressful life events or difficulties occurred, a supportive relationship protected women from depression. However, a two-stage prospective study showed that 40 per cent of relationships, which were reported to be supportive at the first stage, did not prove to be supportive when stressful life events or difficulties actually occurred. Women let down in this way were particularly vulnerable to depression.

Experimental studies

Although randomized control trials are considered to be the Rolls-Royce of designs for assessing the effectiveness of an intervention, investigators are not necessarily publishing more of them. A survey of major journals by two epidemiologists (Fletcher and Fletcher, 1979) suggested that the reverse is true. This may partially be due to constraints of time and money.

Several experiments have been cited in previous chapters. Burke et al.'s (1991) study is a clear example of when a trial is needed to test whether children with otitis do better if given antibiotics. A second example of an important randomized trial was the study by Hollyman et al. (1988) on the effectiveness of amitryptyline in treating depressed patients in general practice.

If is difficult to implement trials to test different ways of delivering primary care. Roland et al. (1986) and Ridsdale et al. (1989) tried to test the effect of time available for consultations on the communication between doctors and patients by arbitrarily allocating patients to surgeries with different appointment intervals. This had the advantage of eliminating the confounding factor of doctors' characteristics which had affected Hughes' (1983) study describing the effects of different appointment times in different practices.

In our study (Ridsdale et al., 1989), it was difficult for the doctors to vary their behaviour in the short time-scale of the study, during which the appointment time available was changed on a weekly basis. It was my subjective impression that the doctors might have changed their consultation behaviour more if they had been given more time to adjust to longer or shorter booking intervals. Even though our practice did increase the time available in consultations after the study was over, the effect could not be tested subsequently. In the long run, other factors in our practice changed too, such as the introduction of the computer to the consulting room. So trying to make experiments work in complex social circumstances is difficult.

Sometimes the opportunity occurs to make a 'natural experiment', where measurements have already been made and then a phenomenon occurs which is believed to affect the subjects' characteristics. For example, Hemenway et al. (1990) measured the activities of doctors in an American clinic before and after the method of remuneration was restructured. The investigators found that when bonuses rewarded increased numbers of tests, significantly more tests were undertaken in the follow-up year. The restructuring of remuneration for cervical screening in the NHS similarly seemed to be associated with a shift in clinical activity towards screening (Reid et al., 1991).

The stage of development of a discipline, and the type of discipline, affects any judgement readers make about the appropriateness of a research design. Very often, a combination of designs and methods will complement each other in making sense of a particular topic.

Other aspects of methodology

When assessing the methods used, readers also need to ask:

1. Is the connection between ideas or concepts and the instruments used, for example, questionnaires, made clear?
2. Is the relationship between the concepts and the measures used to represent them plausible?
3. Are the questionnaires or other instruments used appropriate and previously tested in general practice?

The relationship between ideas and the instruments used to measure them is not always straightforward, especially in general practice, where instruments have only recently been developed, tested and described (Wilkin et al., 1992). When Burke et al. (1991) wanted to know if patients with acute red ear did better on antibiotics, they chose a number of outcomes: duration of fever and crying, analgesic consumption, absence from school and 'treatment failure' where a second antibiotic was required. Readers may put different values on each of these outcomes. Where measurement is difficult, and this is particularly true for children, using several outcome measures may be necessary.

Measuring patient-centredness from audiotaped consultations is extremely difficult, and relating it to plausible outcomes even more so. In this context, Henbest and Stewart (1990) were brave to try to relate interviewing style to process and outcome variables, for example, the doctor's ascertainment of the reason for the patient attending and the resolution of patient concerns. Until instruments are developed, agreed and tested repeatedly, every study of this kind must be seen as a one-off. But they are nonetheless a necessary step towards the development of something better in the future.

4. Is the population and the population sample defined and recognizably similar to that of patients seen in general practice?
5. Were the definitions used when recruiting practices/patients clearly stated, with inclusion and exclusion criteria?
6. Was the sample size sufficient to answer the questions posed? And was this specified in advance?

This last criterion ideally requires investigators to state the critical effect that a new intervention would need to achieve in order for it to be judged clinically better than a placebo, or better than the best alternative treatment. They can then consult a statistical manual to find the sample size they would need in order to demonstrate this effect at a statistically significant level (Kraemer and Thiemann, 1989).

A good example of investigators describing this process was provided by Burke *et al.* (1991). It is likely that in some studies samples or subgroups will be too small, especially when the effect of an intervention is also too small for differences to be statistically significant. This is often a problem in general practice studies. In testing the efficiency of antibiotics for otitis in children, Burke *et al.* chose a sample size sufficient to identify a difference of between 15 per cent and 30 per cent in these outcomes with a power of 0.80. When testing the same hypothesis, Van Buchem *et al.* (1981) started with a similar sample size. They then divided the sample into not two, but four, subgroups which were each treated differently. Under these circumstances, it was less likely that they would identify significant differences between the groups.

When the critical effect of an intervention is small, even national studies may be inconclusive. For example, a national study of the role of aspirin in reducing stroke after transient ischaemic attacks yielded inconclusive results (UK-TIA Study Group, 1988). Only by a meta-analysis of all available studies (Antiplatelet Trialists' Collaboration, 1988) was it possible to demonstrate a statistically significant effect.

7. If this is a randomized control trial to what extent:
   i. are concurrent rather than historical controls used?
   ii. is the method of allocation described?
   iii. is the treatment well defined?
   iv. are the criteria for defining outcome defined and appropriate?

Many outcomes are really measures of process. For example, clofibrate reduces blood lipids but does not reduce total mortality in treated hyperlipidemic patients. A larger proportion of treated patients died than patients in the comparison group (Report of the Committee of Principal Investigators, 1990).

8. Were therapists and those who measured outcome 'blind' as to which patients were in the treatment group and which were in the comparison group?

This is often a difficult requirement to meet, especially in small studies where a GP may both undertake an intervention and evaluate its effect. A study by Johnstone and Goldberg (1976) measured the effectiveness of screening for psychological distress using a questionnaire. The doctor who identified and treated patients and the comparison group, also evaluated its effect. This problem is not unique to general practice. The outcomes of many new hospital-based procedures were often initially measured and described by

Critical appraisal

the same medical or surgical team. Those who have tried to replicate their innovative work have sometimes not been able to demonstrate the same beneficial effect. Where this has been done and reported, it may enhance the credibility readers attach to the results.

9. If a study involved patients, is there reference to approval having been given by the relevant local ethical committee? This process of gaining approval is complicated for GPs, who may have to submit plans to committees most of whose members have little knowledge or experience of primary care. If it is a multi-centre study, this process may need to be repeated several times. Committees aim at ensuring that patients are informed about the necessary details of the research, and of their right not to participate without prejudice to their future care. Ethical committees also require researchers to specify how they will protect patients' confidentiality.

Results

The critical reader will need to know to what extent:

1. was the response rate satisfactory? Were drop-outs well described, and how did they differ from responders?
A high response rate may be particularly difficult to obtain if doctors are the subjects of a study. The national workload studies have only achieved response rates of 58 per cent (DHSS/GMSC, 1987). In collecting characteristics of patients most investigators aim for a 70 per cent response rate at least.

2. are the tables and figures well presented and easy to understand?
Those who do not handle numerical data may tend to avoid looking at tables. This is a shame, as tables often give a different picture to that described in the text. Figures, like histograms, are often easier for readers to cope with, but unfortunately they are more expensive to print. Their omission frequently reduces the clarity of the text.

3. are the statistical tests appropriately applied?
It is unfortunate that statistics are usually taught in the early years of medical school, with almost no subsequent reinforcement. At this early stage, their relevance is often not appreciated by students. Altman (1994) has described the perverse, and perhaps defensive, pride with which doctors admit that they 'don't know anything about statistics'.

4. were confidence intervals used rather than simple 'p' values?
These are generally required by the *British Medical Journal* since a

series of papers describing the techniques were written by Gardner and Altman (1989). The production of a range of values around an average imparts the flavour of notions of confidence and probability, which is what statistics are about, rather than their being about arbitrary cut-off levels for defining significance.

5. was the difference in outcomes sufficient to be clinically important if statistically significant differences were found?

As pointed out earlier, Burke *et al.* (1991) chose several outcomes to test the efficacy of antibiotics on children with red ear. Readers can decide, or even discuss with their patients, how important an outcome such as one day more or less of crying is. In the light of this information, some parents may choose no treatment on behalf of their children, whilst others may choose antibiotics.

6. was a failure to find statistically significant differences due to an inadequate sample size? If the sample size was too small, as frequently occurs when analyzing small subgroups, did the authors point this out?

It is worth emphasizing that, contrary to widespread belief, theories are not proved using conventional statistical techniques. Null theories, for example, that a placebo has no different effect than an active agent, are falsified.

7. assuming that the paper described the results of a randomized control trial,
   i. were the other characteristics of patients who were treated and those in comparison groups comparable? This provides a second check on the effectiveness of randomization procedures.
   ii. were all the subjects followed up, and were they analyzed according to the intention to treat them?

All subjects can rarely be persuaded to stay in a study; this was so in the study of anti-depressants by Hollyman *et al.* (1988). It is important to know how drop-outs differed in their characteristics between groups, and if patients changed groups, as this will bias the results.

Discussion

To what extent:

1. does the discussion demonstrate an awareness of the methodological limitations of the study design and acknowledge any difficulties encountered in carrying out the study?

No study is without difficulties, but if they are identified and described, this truthfulness may increase the reader's confidence.

2. are the conclusions drawn justified by the data presented?
3. do the authors compare and contrast their findings with previously published evidence, both supporting and conflicting?
4. do the authors speculate appropriately, but not too far beyond the evidence provided by the study? Could there be 'prejudice in search of data', and/or could the same data be interpreted differently?

To what extent are these criteria applicable?

All the points on a checklist will not be applicable to each individual paper. An analogy lies in the structure and techniques described for appraising the consultation. GPs will know about the models and skills that have been described by Balint (1957), Byrne and Long (1976), Pendleton *et al.* (1984) and Neighbour (1987). They will not be able to apply all the models to each consultation, but ideally they might apply appropriate models and skills according to the type of problem presented to them. Similarly, different types of evidence will need to be appraised in the most relevant way.

How to learn

Balint groups focussed their discussion on patients who presented problems during the consultation. Groups can learn how to analyze papers in a similar way. My experience is that group members can contribute cumulatively and so identify the strengths and weaknesses of a paper. They can figure out how the results fit or fail to fit in with their experience and decide whether the evidence presented will change their attitudes or practice.

References

Altman, D. G. (1994) The scandal of poor medical research. *British Medical Journal 308:* 283–284.
Anon (1965) The reasons for writing. *British Medical Journal:* 870–872.
Antiplatelet Trialists' Collaboration (1988) Secondary prevention of vascular disease by prolonged anti-platelet treatment. *British Medical Journal 296:* 320–331.
Balint, M. (1957) *The Doctor, his Patient and the Illness.* London: Tavistock.
Beale, N. & Nethercott, S. (1985) Job-loss and family morbidity: A study of a factory closure. *Journal of the Royal College of General Practitioners 35:* 510–514.
Beale, N. & Nethercott, S. (1986) Job-loss and health – the influence of age and previous morbidity. *Journal of the Royal College of General Practitioners 36:* 261–264.

Bosanquet, N. & Leese, B. (1988) Family doctors and innovation in general practice. *British Medical Journal 296:* 1576–1580.

Brown, G. W. & Harris, T. O. (1978) *Social Origins of Depression.* Andover: Tavistock Publications.

Brown, G. W., Andrews, B., Harris, T., Adler, Z. & Bridge, L. (1986) Social support, self-esteem and depression. *Psychological Medicine 16:* 813–831.

Burke, P., Bain, J., Robinson, D. & Dunleavy, J. (1991) Acute red ear in children: Controlled trial of non-antibiotic treatment in general practice. *British Medical Journal 303:* 558–562.

Butler, J. R. & Calnan, M. W. (1987) List sizes and use of time in general practice. *British Medical Journal 295:* 1383–1386.

Byrne, P. & Long, B. (1976) *Doctors Talking to Patients.* London: HMSO.

Calnan, M. W. (1988) Images of general practice: The perceptions of the doctor. *Social Science and Medicine 27:* 579–586.

Calnan, M. W. & Butler, J. R. (1988) The economy of time in general practice: an assessment of the influence of list size. *Social Science and Medicine 26:* 435–441.

Calnan, M. W., Groenewegan, P. P. & Hutten, J. (1992) Professional reimbursement and management of time in general practice: An international comparison. *Social Science and Medicine 35:* 207–216.

Coulter, A. & Baldwin, A. (1987) Surveys of population coverage in cervical cancer screening in the Oxford region. *Journal of the Royal College of General Practitioners 37:* 441–443.

Department of Health and Social Security/General Medical Services Committee (1987) *General Medical Practitioners' Workload. A Report Prepared for the Doctors' and Dentists' Review Body (1985/6).* London: DHSS.

Ellman, R. & Chamberlain, J. (1984) Improving the effectiveness of cervical cancer screening. *Journal of the Royal College of General Practitioners 34:* 537–542.

Fletcher, R. & Fletcher, S. (1979) Clinical research in general medical journals. *New England Journal of Medicine 301:* 180–183.

Gardner, M. J. & Altman, D. G. (1989) *Statistics with Confidence. Confidence Intervals and Statistical Guidelines.* London: BMJ.

Haynes, R. B., Mulrow, C. D., Huth, E. J., Altman, D. G. & Gardner, M. J. (1990) More informative abstracts revisited. *Annals of Internal Medicine 113:* 69–76.

Hemenway, D., Killen, A., Cashman, S., Parks, C. L. & Bicknell, W. J. (1990) Physicians' responses to financial incentives: Evidence from a for-profit ambulatory care centre. *New England Journal of Medicine 322:* 1059–1063.

Henbest, R. J. & Stewart, M. (1990) Patient-centredness in the consultation: Does it really make a difference. *Family Practice 7:* 28–33.

Hollyman, J. A., Freeling, P., Paykel, E. S., Bhat, A. & Sedgwick, P. (1988) Double-blind placebo-controlled trial of amitriptyline among depressed patients in general practice. *Journal of the Royal College of General Practitioners 38:* 393–397.

Horder, J., Bosanquet, N. & Stocking, B. (1986) Ways of influencing the behaviour of general practitioners. *Journal of the Royal College of General Practitioners 36:* 517–521.

Hughes, D. (1983) Consultation length and outcome in two group general practices. *Journal of the Royal College of General Practitioners* 33: 143–147.
Johnstone, A. & Goldberg, D. (1976) Psychiatric screening in general practice: A controlled trial. *The Lancet i:* 605–608.
Kraemer, H. C. & Thiemann, S. (1989) *How Many Subjects?* Newbury Park: Sage Publications.
Morgan, M. & Watkins, C. J. (1988) Managing hypertension: Beliefs and responses to medication among cultural groups. *Sociology of Health and Illness* 10: 561–578.
Neighbour, R. (1987) *The Inner Consultation.* Lancaster: MTP Press Limited.
Norton, P. G., Stuart, M., Tudivert, F. Bass, M. J., Dunn, E. V. (eds) (1991) *Primary Care Research: Traditional and Innovative Approaches.* Newbury Park: Sage Publications.
Pendleton, D., Schofield, T., Tate, P. & Havelock, B. (1984) *The Consultation: An Approach to Learning and Teaching.* Oxford: Oxford University Press.
Reid, G. S., Robertson, A. J., Bissett, C., Smith, J., Waugh, N. & Halkerston, R. (1991) Cervical screening in Perth and Kinross since the introduction of the new contract. *British Medical Journal* 303: 447–450.
Report of the Committee of Principal Investigators (1980) WHO co-operative trial on primary prevention of ischemic heart disease using clofibrate to lower serum cholesterol: Mortality follow-up. *The Lancet ii:* 379.
Ridsdale, L., Carruthers, M., Morris, R. & Ridsdale, J. (1989) Study of the effect of time availability on the consultation. *Journal of the Royal College of General Practitioners* 39: 488–491.
Roland, M. O., Bartholomew, J., Courtenay, M. J. F., Morris, R. W. & Morrell, D. C. (1986) The 'five-minute' consultation: effect of time constraint on verbal communication. *British Medical Journal* 292: 874–876.
Sackett, D. L., Haynes, R. B. & Tugwell, P. (1985) *Clinical Epidemiology: A Basic Science for Clinical Medicine.* Boston/Toronto: Little Brown and Company.
Scambler, G. (1989) *Epilepsy.* London: Tavistock/Routledge.
UK-TIA Study Group (1988) United Kingdom transient ischaemic attack (UK-TIA) Aspirin trial: Interim results. *British Medical Journal* 296: 316–320.
Van Buchem, F. L., Dunk, J. H. M. & Van't Hof, M. A. (1981) Therapy of acute otitis media: myringotomy, antibiotics, or neither? A double blind study in children. *The Lancet ii:* 883–887.
Wilkin, D., Hallam, L. & Doggett, M.-A. (1992) *Measures of Need and Outcome for Primary Care.* Oxford: Oxford Medical Publications.

14

A Critical Appraisal of the Literature on Tiredness

> The following morning I got up early. One of the journals which is distributed free to general practitioners had asked me to write a summary of the literature on tiredness. As it was a topic on which I had done a research project and reviewed the literature, I believed I could meet the journal's deadline which was only a week away (Ridsdale, 1994).

Introduction

In the previous chapter, a framework was outlined for appraising papers. One way for practitioners to develop their skills further is to imagine a journal editor has asked for a review of the literature for a particular topic. A busy clinician will not have a lot of time to do this, so he or she might first think of the key words authors might use when writing up research on this topic and then ask a librarian to do a literature search using these key words. The clinician should then sift through the literature, at the same time keeping in mind his or her own clinical experience, and the criteria for judging the papers' validity and their usefulness in primary care. This chapter will provide an example of this process by pointing out the strengths and weaknesses of the literature on tiredness, in the context of GPs confronted by patients who complain of this problem.

Is it important?

Before even looking at an article on a particular issue, GPs will want to know to what extent this topic is important or relevant for their work. How can they judge what is important and what criteria can be helpful? The problem might be considered important if it had a high prevalence in the community. The results of a descriptive survey could be a useful source of such information. Hannay (1978) and the Health Promotion Research Trust (1987) described the frequency of individuals complaining of tiredness in the community. The symptom of tiredness was a frequent problem, and Hannay found it was the second most common physical symptom after respiratory symptoms.

However, a problem occurring frequently in the community does not necessarily mean that it is important for general practitioners. To a certain extent, doctors will evaluate whether a problem is important by the frequency with which they see it in their consulting rooms. Morrell (1972) asked all the doctors in his practice to record the symptoms presented to them over the course of 1 year. He found that of the new symptoms presented, cough was the most frequent, whilst a loss of energy or tiredness was the fourteenth most frequent symptom. Fatigue is therefore less frequently seen or reported in the consulting room than in the community. It is not one of the most common symptoms presented, but neither is it seen rarely.

Are the questions already answered?

So far as the topic of fatigue is concerned, there has been comparatively little research. Many questions remain unanswered or have not even been posed. So at this point of development of the topic, descriptive studies are useful and appropriate. They may help to identify future questions and to test instruments that can be used to answer these and other questions in the future.

Is the site similar enough to general practice?

Perhaps the most important and difficult area for general practitioners is to look at the study environment of the research done on fatigue and to decide whether it is similar enough to their own area of experience for them to use the evidence in their own practice. Goldberg and Huxley (1992) have described the stages at which measurements can be made of patients' characteristics on the pathway from the community to psychiatric care. They described five levels and four filters, shown in Table 14.1.

These sites and filters are equally applicable when examining research on patients with fatigue. Some studies of patients at levels 1 and 3 have already been described; Hannay (1978) and the Health Promotion Research Trust (1987) measured the prevalence of fatigue in the community, and Morrell (1972) measured the frequency with which this symptom was presented to GPs.

Table 14.1 *The pathway to psychiatric care.*

Level 1	The community
	1st filter (illness behaviour)
Level 2	Attenders in primary care
	2nd filter (ability to detect disorder)
Level 3	Mental illness identified by doctors
	3rd filter (referral to mental illness services)
Level 4	Mental illness services
	4th filter (admission to psychiatric beds)
Level 5	Psychiatric in-patients

Studies have been done at other points along the pathway to medical care. For example, Valdini *et al.* (1988) and David *et al.* (1990) measured the prevalence of fatigue among patients in the general practice waiting room (level 2). The advantage of this kind of study is that potentially all the patients who attended the doctor were assessed, and variability in selection or identification by doctors working in the consulting room was eliminated. However, the disadvantage of identifying patients in this location is that it is difficult to know what can be extrapolated that will affect clinical practice. Patients sitting in the waiting room may have a whole range of clinical conditions, for example virus infections, and these may be associated with tiredness. This is less of a problem for doctors in terms of differential diagnosis, when fatigue is sometimes classified as a 'supporting' symptom. The study by David *et al.* coincided with a winter epidemic of flu (Curwen *et al.*, 1990), so it is particularly difficult to know what general practitioners might extrapolate from their results to normal practice.

At the other end of the pathway to medical care, Yousef *et al.* (1988) reported that a group of patients referred with post-viral fatigue syndrome were more likely to have evidence of Coxsackie B viruses than a comparison group. On the basis of this, some GPs began to request Coxsackie B virus tests on patients with fatigue. However, it is quite difficult from reading the paper to be sure how these patients were selected, or how each of the patients was selected who formed the comparison group. Without specific details of this kind which relate to the study environment and recruitment criteria, it is not possible for general practitioners to know whether they can extrapolate from the evidence to primary care.

Methods

Is the design appropriate?

Observational studies
In the process of learning about a particular topic, different types of study designs will yield different and potentially useful data. Useful descriptive studies have already been cited by Hannay (1978), Morrell (1972) and the Health Promotion Research Trust (1987). This is quantitative work which required the investigators to define what they were looking at in advance and then to measure the numbers of patients who fell into each category. In virtually all the studies, more women were found to be fatigued than men.

An alternative approach might be to ask what the experience of fatigue meant to these people in a more open-ended way. Oakley (1974) interviewed a small group of housewives on several occasions about the nature of their work and its advantages and disadvantages for them. She was able to provide a detailed account of their working conditions and the lack of boundaries they experienced between one activity and another. The relative autonomy, but continuing responsibility, experienced by housewives was eloquently described using this qualitative approach.

Popay (1992) added to the perspective provided by this in-depth approach by interviewing a small group of men and women in London over the course of 1 year. She was able to compare and contrast the roles of parents and their sense of responsibility for their young children. She combined reports of the perceptions and experiences of these adults with a detailed analysis of data from the Health Promotion Research Trust (1987). This showed that women were particularly likely to report fatigue when they had children under 6 years of age.

Retrospective studies
A question that doctors will ask and want to know the answer to when assessing patients with fatigue is: what are the causes likely to be? These questions were posed, and some evidence has been derived from retrospective studies by Morrison (1980) and Sugarman and Berg (1984). These American investigators examined the case notes of patients who had been classified as fatigued at the end of the consultation, in order to decide on the productivity of investigations and the diagnosis achieved. However, any doctor who has examined case notes will know that it is difficult to categorize data from doctors' notes when, at the time of recording, the doctors were unaware that a study was going to be undertaken. The tests requested by these doctors will have varied considerably. Even their use of the category fatigue at the end of the consultation

will probably have been extremely variable. In the General Practice Morbidity Survey (RCGP, OPCS, DHSS, 1986), general practitioners did vary widely in their use of the category fatigue in a way which was similar to their variable use of psychological illness categories. Those doctors who are reluctant to accept uncertainty at the end of the clinical reasoning process may be more likely to apply a specific diagnosis, whereas other doctors may be comfortable to categorize patients symptomatically when no definitive diagnosis has been made.

Morrison (1980) found that married women were more likely to be diagnosed as fatigued than their single counterparts. This finding might fit well with Oakley's (1974) and Popay's (1992) qualitative studies of the work and role responsibilities of mothers of young children. However, Morrison also reported that physical diagnoses were more likely to be made by doctors working in the private sector and psychological diagnoses by doctors who worked in academic centres. Both doctors and patients may attach a stigma to psychological labels. This systematic bias in labelling reduces the reader's confidence when the researcher subsequently tries to relate the social characteristics of patients to the diagnoses applied by doctors.

Prospective studies
Miller *et al.* (1991) used a prospective case-control study to test the hypothesis that Coxsackie B virus is associated with the fatigue syndrome. Patients presenting with fatigue were tested for the virus, and matched controls were obtained from the same general practitioner. About a quarter of patients in both groups were positive for Coxsackie B virus. Results in both groups showed a strong seasonal variation. When these data are compared to those of Yousef *et al.* (1988), who had suggested that Coxsackie B was a likely cause of fatigue, the different findings underline the importance of defining the criteria for selecting cases and the comparison group in advance.

In order to provide more information about the predictive yield of laboratory tests and the likely diagnosis made, a group of GPs (Ridsdale *et al.*, 1993; 1994) observed patients who presented with a main symptom of fatigue in four British practices. In this study, the yield of a standard group of tests could be estimated and the natural history of the condition observed. Evidence of this kind about the natural history may be useful before controlled trials of particular forms of therapy are undertaken.

Experiments
Although treatments for fatigue have not been systematically assessed, there have been some natural experiments and trials which provide some insights as to the cause. Imboden *et al.* (1961;

1972) administered psychological questionnaires to a group of 600 employees 3 to 6 months before an influenza epidemic. At the time of the epidemic, 26 persons reported sick to the dispensary and a subgroup of 12 had not recovered 3 to 6 weeks later. Their most frequent complaint was fatigue. This symptomatic subgroup had significantly higher scores on their psychological questionnaires, suggesting that they had an emotional disturbance prior to the flu epidemic. The number of individuals involved was very small, but the evidence lends support to the idea that a pre-existing psychological problem may be associated with slower recovery from a reported infection, with persistent fatigue as a symptom.

Cohen *et al.* (1991) asked a group of healthy volunteers to complete psychological questionnaires about perceived life events and distress, and then gave them a measured dose of respiratory viruses and quarantined them in the Common Cold Unit. They found the rates of both respiratory infection and clinical colds increased in a dose response manner with increases in the degree of pre-recorded psychological distress. Both these studies identify a factor which seems to have a negative effect, and they contribute evidence about a possible causal sequence involving psychological distress and impaired immunity or delayed recovery from viral infections.

Ideas and measurement

The connection between concepts and the instruments used to measure them is an extremely important and difficult thing to evaluate. From their own personal experience and their knowledge of the literature, clinicians are likely to agree that there is a plausible case for a relationship existing between fatigue and psychological distress. What is not clear from the literature is whether:

1. fatigue causes psychological distress;
2. psychological distress causes fatigue;
3. both sequences occur; or
4. the two states come into existence due to some antecedent or intervening phenomena like impaired immunity.

How can these concepts be measured? As far as psychological distress or illness is concerned, it is very difficult to measure the concept as long as psychiatrists disagree about how it should be defined. Despite being aware of this conceptual murkiness, psychiatric researchers have developed standardized instruments to measure psychological illness in general practice. A labour-intensive, and therefore expensive, method of measurement is to use a standard research interview. A self-rating questionnaire such as the General Health Questionnaire is a less expensive alternative. Goldberg and Williams (1988) have reviewed the literature on the use of this instrument, which has been extensively tested in general practice.

However, when it comes to measuring fatigue, it is much more difficult to find a measure which has been repeatedly tested. The fatigue questionnaire developed by Wessely and Powell (1989), tested by Chalder et al. (1993) and applied by David et al. (1990) and Pawlikowska et al. (1994), is the best currently available. It is an instrument which is still in the process of development rather than necessarily being the final product, and studies which have used it, including my own, could also be seen as means rather than ends in the process of developing reliable measures.

Is the population sampled similar?

It is particularly important for general practitioners to look at the definition of the population sample in more detail when studies are reported from other countries. For example, Kroenke et al. (1988) entitled one of their papers 'Chronic fatigue in primary care'. This has been cited by British psychiatric researchers (Lynch et al., 1991) as though the study originated in primary care. The location where patients were recruited to this American study was described by the authors as a teaching hospital, including an internal medicine clinic providing care for adults with chronic medical problems and an acute care clinic providing care on a walk-in basis for minor illness. The term 'primary care' seems to have a different meaning in North America. British researchers and clinicians need to be aware of this alternative meaning in order not to be misled.

Similarly, definitions of the control groups used in American studies need to be scrutinized carefully. Patients in North America do not register with one general practitioner, and so other patients on the list cannot be used for the purposes of comparison. Studies of fatigue reported by Valdini et al. (1988) and Cathebras et al. (1992) used other patients attending the doctors as the comparison group. But if the intention of a study is to describe the characteristics of patients with fatigue, some differences will be lost if attenders with similar characteristics are used for the purposes of comparison. Three times as many women as men complain of fatigue as their main problem (Ridsdale et al., 1993), and three times as many women as men attend the surgery for any given reason (David et al., 1990). A study such as that by Cathebras et al. (1992), which compared patients with fatigue with other attenders, are likely to find, as indeed they did, that there was no gender difference between the two groups.

Was the sample of sufficient size?

Sample size is important even in descriptive studies, but whatever the sample size chosen, the results will be inconclusive for some subgroups. For example, in our study of patients with fatigue, men complained of the symptom three times less frequently than women (Ridsdale et al., 1993). However, when fatigue was the main complaint, the outcome for men was worse at 6 months. As the number of men in the sample was small, this result was not statistically significant. An hypothesis concerning the relationship between gender and the duration of fatigue symptoms could not be tested in any conclusive way without a larger sample size.

Results

Response rates

Investigators generally hope for a response rate of about 70 per cent. Response rates will tend to go down when subjects are required to do more for little perceived gain. Cathebras et al. (1992) asked surgery attenders to be interviewed for 2 hours at the time of seeing a doctor, and 51 per cent agreed to participate. Although the socio-demographic characteristics of the non-responders were found to be similar, the authors could not exclude the possibility that the information provided by the people who were willing to discuss their illness experience with the investigators was not representative of the 49 per cent who were not willing to do so. In our experience of studying patients in Britain using relatively simple questionnaires (Ridsdale et al, 1993), patients were much more likely to respond, and 78 per cent of the inception cohort returned their questionnaires 6 months later. This willingness to participate and respond may have been aided by the NHS system whereby patients are registered with particular doctors who will be responsible for those patients ongoing care.

Are the data understandable?

In attempting to make sense of data which purport to measure complex concepts like psychological distress and fatigue, readers may find themselves bewildered. Even when a standardized questionnaire like the General Health Questionnaire is used, the method of coding will make a considerable difference to the results. Possible responses can be scored in the conventional way described by Goldberg and Williams (1988). This method allocates no points for a symptom being the same or better than usual, and one point for the symptom being worse or much worse than usual. Alternatively, symptoms can be scored using a Lykert scale, which can be used to determine the severity of symptoms using a scale from 0 to 3. The traditional method yields a product that represents the number of symptoms present, but not their severity. The Lykert method produces a larger number, which is influenced by the severity of the symptoms. A Lykert scoring method is also more likely to yield data that conform to a bell-shaped, normal pattern when plotted on frequency distribution. Pawlikowska *et al.* (1994) have illustrated their data in this way. Some statistical manipulations depend on a normal distribution of scores, so the way researchers code and analyze their data is important, and affects their 'findings'. These are complex issues. How they are managed by researchers is important both for themselves and for others who are trying to make sense of the possible relationship, for example, between psychological distress and tiredness.

Data management in the analysis of psychological characteristics may seem, to the uninitiated, like a sophisticated conjuring trick. However, making sense of data from so-called 'hard' laboratory tests is not necessarily more straightforward. In our prospective study of the yield of laboratory tests in patients presenting with fatigue, we initially recorded the results of a standard group of laboratory tests using the laboratories' criteria for abnormality (Ridsdale *et al.*, 1993). Laboratories usually derive their parameters statistically to generate results that will be reported as within or outside the normal range. However, it is transparently clear to all clinicians that results reported as abnormal are not necessarily clinically important, and that if enough tests are done patients will be found to have an abnormality by what is sometimes called 'chance'. In our study, it also transpired that one laboratory had not used a reliable method for an important test used for the study, the monospot test. This laboratory found that, for several years, it had been generating a higher than expected level of abnormalities. Half way through the study the laboratory abandoned the use of this particular testing method.

Given the limitations of standard laboratory tests, we asked the general practitioners in the study to answer the question: which laboratory tests yielded clinically important results when taken in conjunction with other data? This assessment depended on a clinical and subjective judgement made by doctors, and these judgements are likely to have varied from one doctor to another. When the history, physical examination, laboratory results and outcome are taken together as criteria for making judgements it is likely, as Sackett *et al.* (1985) have pointed out, that doctors will vary a great deal. In arriving at a judgement about a diagnosis, the problem of inter-rater differences exists as much for hospital doctors like cardiologists and radiologists as it does for general practitioners.

Discussion

It has already been suggested that the space allowed for the introduction and discussion is often too small for authors to place their findings in context, especially in biomedical journals. It may also be extremely difficult for investigators to do this immediately after analyzing their work. For this reason, readers may often rely on editorials or discussion papers to see evidence put into context.

However, writers who do point out the problems they experienced during a study and who resist the temptation to make grandiose claims for their findings are more likely to be believed. The issue of veracity is extremely difficult to describe without invoking the wrath of other investigators. So researchers tend to talk to each other about the credibility of their colleagues without putting this in print. It is clearly very difficult to strike a balance between the bland incremental approach often found in discussion sections, and the vitriolic excesses which make the letters to the editor such spicy reading.

The difference in the style of writing between the humanities and the sciences is greatest when it comes to a willingness to express criticism. In the sciences, investigators are mutually dependent in that they depend on their colleagues' judgements about their work when they make grant applications and when they submit their papers to journals. One can only speculate that this and other factors may limit the amount of published criticism.

A lack of balanced criticism in scientific journals does, however, diminish the confidence of readers who are practitioners. Similarly, clinicians' tendency to stick together and not criticize colleagues, even when it is justified, may diminish the confidence of patients. There are some doctors few of us would trust our family with. There are also some researchers who do not inspire the confidence of their colleagues. It seems unacceptable that patients and readers will only be able to recognize a consistent incompetent by careful scrutiny or by having inside information.

Readers should not conclude from this that most papers reporting research can be divided up in a simple yes/no way. Most papers have strengths and weaknesses, and the investigators will have worked long and hard to produce their work. It is important for referees and reviewers to bear both points in mind. Critical reviews need not involve the metaphorical sharpening of knives. The process should be seen as a way of drawing out useful answers and asking new questions. Viewed in this way, the reviewer can be seen as having a creative, redescribing role.

References

Cathebras, P. J., Robbins, J. M., Kirmayer, L. J. & Hayton, B. C. (1992) Fatigue in primary care: Prevalence, psychiatric co-morbidity, illness behaviour, and outcome. *Journal of General Internal Medicine* 7: 276–286.

Chalder, T., Berelowitz, G., Pawlikowska, T., Watts, L., Wessely, S., Wright, D. et al. (1993) Development of a fatigue scale. *Journal of Psychosomatic Research* 37: 147–153.

Cohen, S., Tyrrell, D. A. J. & Smith, A. P. (1991) Psychological stress and susceptibility to the common cold. *New England Journal of Medicine* 325: 606–612.

Curwen, M., Dunnell, K. & Ashley, J. (1990) Hidden influenza deaths. *British Medical Journal* 300: 896.

David, A., Pelosi, A., McDonald, E., Stephens, D., Ledger, D., Rathbone, R. & Mann, A. (1990) Tired, weak, or in need of rest: Fatigue among general practice attenders. *British Medical Journal* 301: 1199–1202.

Goldberg, D. & Huxley, P. (1992) *Common Mental Disorders: A Biosocial Model*. London: Routledge.

Goldberg, D. & Williams, P. (1988) *A User's Guide to the General Health Questionnaire*. Windsor: NFER-Nelson Publishing Company Limited.

Hannay, D. R. (1978) Symptom prevalence in the community. *Journal of the Royal College of General Practitioners* 28: 492–493.

Health Promotion Research Trust (1987) *The Health and Lifestyle Survey*. London: Health Promotion Research Trust.

Imboden, J. B. (1972) Psychosocial determinants of recovery. *Advances in Psychosomatic Medicine* 8: 142–155.

Imboden, J. B. Canter, A. & Cluff, L. E. (1961) Convalescence from influenza. *Archives of Internal Medicine* 108: 393–399.

Kroenke, K., Wood, D. R., Mangelsdorff, A. D., Mieer, N. J. & Powell, J. B. (1988) Chronic fatigue in primary care: Prevalence, patient characteristics, and outcome. *Journal of the American Medical Association* 260: 929–935.

Lynch, S., Seth, R. & Montgomery, S. (1991) Antidepressant therapy in the chronic fatigue syndrome. *British Journal of Medical Practice* 41: 339–342.

Miller, N. A., Carmichael, H. A., Calder, B. D., Behan, P. O., Bell, E. J., McCartney, R. A. & Hall, F. C. (1991) Antibody to Coxsackie B virus in diagnosing postviral fatigue syndrome. *British Medical Journal* 302: 140–143.

Morrell, D. C. (1972) Symptom interpretation in general practice. *Journal of the Royal College of General Practitioners* 22: 297–309.

Morrison, J. D. (1980) Fatigue as a presenting complaint in family practice. *Journal of Family Practice* 10: 795–801.

Oakley, A. (1974) *A Sociology of Housework*. London: Pitman.

Pawlikowska, T., Chalder, T., Hirsch, S. R., Wallace, P., Wright, D. J. M. & Wessely, S. L. (1994) Population based study of fatigue and psychological distress. *British Medical Journal* 308: 763–766.

Popay, J. (1992) My health is all right, but I'm just tired all the time: women's experience of ill health. In: Roberts, H. (ed) *Women's Health Matters*, pp. 99–120. London: Routledge.

Ridsdale, L. (1994) Tired all the time. *Well Women Team* 15: 12–13.

Ridsdale, L., Evans, A., Jerrett, W., Mandalia, S., Osler, K. & Vora, H. (1993)

Patients with fatigue in general practice: A prospective study. *British Medical Journal* 307: 103–106.

Ridsdale, L., Evans, A., Jerrett, W., Mandalia, S., Osler, K. & Vora, H. (1994) Patients who consult with tiredness: frequency of consultation, perceived causes of tiredness and its association with psychological distress. *British Journal of General Practice* 44: 413–416.

Royal College of General Practitioners, Offices of Population Censuses and Surveys, and Department of Health and Social Security (1986) *Morbidity Statistics from General Practices. Third National Study, 1981–1982.* London: HMSO.

Sackett, D. L., Haynes, R. B. & Tugwell, P. (1985) *Clinical Epidemiology: A Basic Science for Clinical Medicine.* Boston: Little Brown and Company.

Sugarman, J. R. & Berg, A. O. (1984) Evaluation of fatigue in a family practice. *Journal of Family Practice* 19: 643–647.

Valdini, A. F., Steinhardt, S., Valicenti, J. & Jaffe, A. (1988) A one-year follow-up of fatigue patients. *Journal of Family Practice* 26: 33–38.

Wessely, S. & Powell, R. (1989) Fatigue syndromes: A comparison of chronic 'post viral' fatigue with neuromuscular and affective disorders. *Journal of Neurology, Neuro-surgery, and Psychiatry* 52: 940–948.

Yousef, G. E., Bell, E. J., Mann, G. F., Murugesan, V., Smith, D. G. & McCartney, R. A. (1988) Chronic enterovirus infection in patients with postviral fatigue syndrome. *The Lancet i:* 146–150.

15

How Do You Know? The Process of Scientific Reasoning

> I went to the local medical centre. A specialist was introduced, the lights were dimmed. For 50 minutes he ran through a series of slides on the topic advertised. When he had finished, the lights went up, and the questions started. The audience of GPs were trying to relate their clinical experience to the evidence that had been presented to them.

Introduction

Scientists, doctors and patients, indeed everyone, are concerned with making sense of what is going on around them. This process involves observing events that have occurred in the past and attributing causal connections between them. By doing this, people can usually convince themselves that what they observe is not necessarily chaotic and random, and that they may be able to predict from their associations something about what is going to happen in the future. Patients and society generally invest scientists and doctors with a special ability to recognize causal connections and predict future events, so it is worth considering the processes whereby this is achieved and to what extent people's confidence in scientific reasoning is justified. This chapter will focus on explanations or models of how scientific reasoning takes place.

I see it, therefore it is: inductivism

Having memorized the requisite number of facts to pass final medical examinations, most doctors say they subsequently learn by

How do you know? The process of scientific reasoning   161

experience. Indeed, general practitioners have reified experiential learning as *the process* by which doctors acquire knowledge. It is claimed that this process of acquiring knowledge enables more experienced practitioners to become even more knowing and skilful.

The assumption that experience is the best teacher is an attractive one. Personal experience has an immediacy which lends it a strong truth value. However, there are problems with inferring causal relationships from our own experience and observations. These will be illustrated by an example.

Patient needs and medical monopolies

During the 1980s, there was a large group practice in a neighbouring community consisting entirely of male partners. The senior partner maintained that the practice had thrived and that the community was well cared for without a woman partner. His junior partners disagreed, and when he retired they recruited a woman to take over his list. Now let us look for the fallacies in the original argument. The practice did thrive with no woman partner, but new doctors could not enter without permission from the Medical Practices Committee, so the practice was a unique provider, or monopoly, in economic terms. As no competitors could enter the market, it is likely that the practice would thrive. Secondly, there was evidence that some pockets of need were not completely met under the old system. In the evening, the local authority used the health centre to provide a family planning service which was staffed by women doctors. The clinics were well attended, suggesting a need which was met within the building, but separately from the group practice.

In Chapter 5, it was noted that men with emotional problems were more likely to consult women partners when they were available in the practice (Boardman, 1987). Unmet demand of this kind is difficult to define and measure, but there is some evidence that emotional distress goes on longer when it goes unrecognized and untreated (Johnstone and Goldberg, 1976). Approximately 4,000 patients commit suicide in England and Wales each year, and the ratio of male to female deaths is 3:1 (OPCS, 1993). The total number of deaths is twice as large as the number of deaths from cervical cancer. It might be argued that it is therefore important to provide at least one woman partner in a practice for men who have emotional problems and who express a preference for confiding this to a female doctor.

These are only arguments. Nevertheless, the senior partner believed what he observed. It was impossible in a fixed social context to test his hypothesis and to distinguish between cause and effect. The continued process of believing something and selectively observing it to occur makes people more and more convinced that their own beliefs are correct. When challenged about their different practices, doctors often put down their differences to 'experience'. But adding up these experiences is inconclusive. As an inductive approach is problematic, it is therefore worth considering some alternatives to inductive reasoning with regard to scientific evidence and practice.

I believe what has not yet been falsified: falsificationism

Observers are selective. What they observe depends on the theories which preceded their observations. People more often see what they believe, rather than believing what they see.

An alternative approach to making sense of what goes on in scientific reasoning is to ignore the initial phase of observation and assume that theories are just imaginative mental creations. Popper (Popper, 1968; Magee, 1982) suggested that scientists may initially invent or imagine relationships between phenomena and that we need not worry about how they derived the associations they propose. The important thing, according to Popper, was that proposed causal associations should be clearly stated and tested. The criterion for a scientific theory, according to Popper, was its testability and its ability to withstand repeated attempts at falsification. Popper acknowledged that some scientific theories could not be tested and would not be falsifiable given the technology available at the time. However, he maintained that theories would, in the long run, be able to be tested. If they were falsified, scientists should abandon them for a better theory. This abandonment should not be regarded as a failure, because all theories are only tentative and provisional explanations. There can be no certainty or absolute truth. Having urged scientists to abandon falsified theories, Popper then qualified this assertion by pointing out that in some cases scientists may need to be tenacious in sustaining their belief in a theory when observations which others claim falsify it are themselves open to question.

Popper's contribution is useful as it rejected a dogmatic approach to scientific knowledge which sought to establish a sense of certainty. It asserted that there are no such things as facts. Popper emphasized that the scientific process consisted of investigators addressing problems with proposed solutions, testing their propositions and moving on, by a process of trial and error, to a preferred theory which could only ever be provisional. He also emphasized the need for scientists to criticize their own work and the duty of seeking out and valuing critical feedback from others (McIntyre and Popper, 1983). In doing this, he prefigured the development of the clinical audit.

How do you know? The process of scientific reasoning

Popper's vision of what scientists were or should be doing has coincided to a great extent with what scientists perceived themselves to be doing in the twentieth century. The model of hypothesis testing and falsification has become a dominant scientific style. Scientists in the medical world like Medawar (1969) and Cochrane (1972) worked independently to develop and champion this approach.

But this method does not necessarily provide clear answers when practitioners want to know what to do. An example is the question of whether to prescribe for earaches or not. British practitioners have reported that they almost always prescribe antibiotics, whereas Dutch doctors reported that they do not generally do so (Froom et al., 1990). Both these groups observe that their patients generally recover from earaches quickly. This experience reinforces their beliefs about cause and effect. Popper's approach ideally requires that scientists explicitly state a causal relationship and put it to the test with a randomized control trial. The proposition would be that children of a certain age with pink eardrums will recover more quickly with an antibiotic, such as amoxycillin, than children treated with what appears to be amoxycillin but which is in fact a placebo.

The scientific process described in Chapters 3 and 13 requires that children be randomly allocated to the two groups so that other causes of a favourable or unfavourable outcome, like age or social class, will not interfere with the result. Neither the children nor their carers should know which child is taking the active agent and which is not. These are the principles of randomization and double-blinding. And the sample size must be of a sufficient size for an important difference in outcome to be statistically detectable (Kraemer and Thiemann, 1991).

Trials like this have been done. In one centre, there were significantly better outcomes among children taking the active agent than were found among the comparison group (Burke et al., 1981). In a study of children with recurrent otitis media reported only a few months later, no significant difference was found in the course of symptoms regardless of whether antibiotics were given or not (Appelman et al., 1991). Practitioners who believed that antibiotics ameliorated the course of otitis media found that their hypothesis had not been falsified. Physicians who believed that antibiotics made no difference also found evidence that did not falsify their belief. Both groups were able to question the methods and observations used to test the hypothesis which they did not favour, and question the observations made. It has been shown in Chapter 13 that research methods and observations are often vulnerable to criticism, and in this context it is difficult to refute an hypothesis decisively.

We know what we agree: a social approach

Kuhn (1970) proposed a criticism of Popper's ideas. He argued that there is no such thing as a language which taps directly into observations. When joining a discipline or profession, scientists learn a language which encompasses a core group of theories, with a protective belt of lesser theories that can be discarded if necessary. Kuhn suggested that once scientists had learnt the language and 'world view' of their own profession, they tend to become conservative, or consensus seeking, and abandon a critical approach. Kuhn's central thesis was that, having learned the language which describes the content of a discipline, scientists confine themselves largely to solving puzzles. They resolve anomalies by making suitable adjustments which leave the core of their theory, or 'paradigm', intact.

Kuhn was particularly concerned with how theories or knowledge change, and with the resistance to change put up by the scientific community. He likened a change in a scientific paradigm to translating a language. A good translation manual for the language of another region and culture should include paragraphs explaining how native speakers of that language view the world. Kuhn claimed that part of learning to translate a language or a theory required learning to describe the world in which the language or theory functioned. Those who have moved from practising in a hospital to practising in the community, or who have learned new languages, will appreciate the difficulties involved in doing this. Kuhn also emphasized the social or conventional nature of theories, and the way in which professionalization led to an unquestioning approach. When confronted by anomalies or counter-instances to their own theories, he suggested that most scientists devise numerous *ad hoc* modifications in order to eliminate conflict.

Kuhn described major belief or theory changes among scientists as being like religious conversions. Doctors who have learned a traditional biophysical approach to medicine have described the acquisition and integration of psychosocial perspectives in general practice as an example of a conversion to a new paradigm (Howie, 1984; McWhinney, 1983). Although this was not a scientific revolution on the scale alluded to by Kuhn, many GPs found the conventional medical model inappropriate and inadequate in the community. When the paradigm failed, some doctors felt confused and disillusioned (Morrell, 1993). They had specialized in physical and biological science since their early teens; the acquisition of the language of social science much later was a difficult but enlightening process.

Kuhn was pessimistic about the way in which most scientists and professionals work. He may have chosen major belief changes as

How do you know? The process of scientific reasoning

examples in order to bolster this view. But GPs will recognize some truth in Kuhn's description of the acquisition of a shared language and values in medicine. Most trainees and GPs have experience of professional groups who generate a cosy, shared view of the world and who are fairly resistant to critical thinking. Moreover, for general practitioners in the United Kingdom, doctors are required contractually to defend their behaviour by doing what, in their place, other doctors would also do. In this way, shared views about shared behaviour are perpetuated and are legally reinforced.

We know what we agree to say: a linguistic approach

When serving an apprenticeship to become members of the medical community, doctors learn a specific language which has accepted meanings and which enables them to function in the medical community. Saussure (1974), a linguist, described an earlier learning process, pointing out that everyone serves an apprenticeship in language as a young child. When acquiring language, children learn and build into their language conventions about values and meanings which are specific to a particular society and its history. There is no automatic relationship between a word and the object or concept it represents. In one country, for example, the object illustrated here will be called 'un arbre' and in another country 'a tree'.

Saussure proposed that language functioned as a collection of necessary conventions that have been adopted by a social group. It is as though a contract has been signed by members of a community about the association between words and the concepts they refer to. New members of a society must serve an apprenticeship in

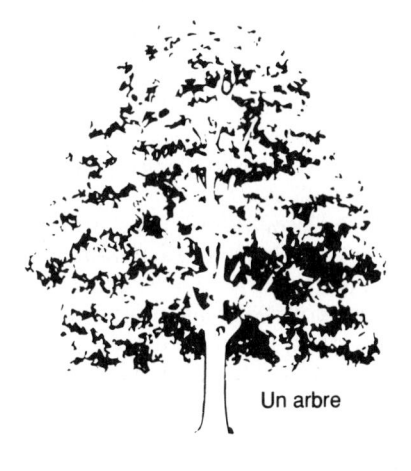

Un arbre

Fig. 15.2 A tree

learning a new system. And when one considers the sum of the efforts required to learn our mother tongue or a new language, it is likely that there will be subsequent resistance to change, although small changes do occur over time. This process may determine what is 'seen' and counted as significant in medical terms also.

Foucault (1981) applied this 'structure of language' approach to the development of psychiatry as a science during the nineteenth century. He claimed that during the nineteenth century, medical practitioners gradually took over the role which had previously been occupied by priests, erecting a science on the site of what had previously been the confession. Psychiatrists and psychoanalysts codified symptoms and signs, but in doing so they introduced prejudices and stereotypes about sexual differences and sexual behaviour, which were then applied as if they were explanatory factors. In place of notions of error, sin, excess or transgression, medical science adopted a concept of the normal versus the pathological. As doctors changed the confession into the consultation, society's values were superimposed on it. *Plus ça change, plus c'est la même chose!*

Foucault claimed that this new scientific language incorporated traditional values. Psychiatrists labelled the objects of their attention. Once labelled, they somehow took on a reality of their own. Pathological types created by the new taxonomy included 'the nervous woman', 'the indifferent mother', 'the frigid wife', 'the homosexual'. Foucault condemned the creation of these labels and the practice of subjecting less powerful groups to treatment.

General practitioners spend hours listening to the problems of families and relationships. It is worth reflecting on Foucault's description of the history of this confessional role. An approach which emphasizes language and meaning may be helpful for understanding the areas where teaching through conventional stereotypes seems to have led to needy groups being 'overlooked'. Three-quarters of those who commit suicide in Britain are men, but Boardman (1987) found that doctors tended to overlook depressive symptoms in men, whereas they found and treated depression significantly more often in women. This process may reflect self-fulfilling expectations which have become engrained in the language and the culture.

Gellner (1992) showed how interdependent language, social values and a scientific approach are in medicine. He argued that language and reasoning are specific to a certain society at a particular time. Placed within this context, reasoning cannot be separated out from society's values. However, our language already incorporates long-lasting contrasting concepts, such as the idea that reason can function independently of cultural influences and the idea that the body can be separated from the mind. The idea that reasoning is dependent on language and the social context may therefore seem

How do you know? The process of scientific reasoning 167

disturbing. In the same way, if doctors are unable to question some of the accepted language and concepts they have inherited, they may not be helping, and may even be harming, their patients.

A pluralist approach

When evaluating the different approaches to scientific reasoning and knowledge, each one can be seen to have its own merits. When choosing between treatments, GPs will rightly look for the results from randomized controlled trials. But it has been emphasized that appraising papers can be as difficult as doing the research in the first place. Authors may not describe their methods clearly, they tend to publish results when the outcome was beneficial and often do not publish 'negative' or inconclusive results. The instruments and outcomes they choose are often not strictly comparable. For this reason the process of gathering information about and critically evaluating different treatments has become a science in itself (Chalmers et al., 1992).

The process of doing systematic meta-analyses and reviews combines the two classical scientific approaches of induction and falsification. Randomized controlled trials were originally set up to test rival hypotheses with a view to falsifying one or the other. But the process of gathering, appraising and adding up the evidence from *all* the studies of one treatment modality is inductive. The sum of the evidence provides increasingly more or less support for rival theories (Howson and Urbach, 1989). Particular causal theories become more or less probable over time. It always remains possible that some observations are wrong and that some theories are wrong. The idea of certainty is an illusion, but in weighing up the probabilities some doctors (and patients) can learn to live and cope with uncertainty. Fromm (1960) and Rorty (1989) described the process whereby people avoid uncertainty by affiliating themselves to leaders or belief systems that claim to embody the absolute truth. It is perhaps this need for certainty which contributes to the success of dogmatic politicians and doctors.

When describing the people GPs see in their surgeries with economic, social and psychological difficulties, the approaches offered by social scientists and linguists are also appropriate. The biographical processes of providing care in a particular subculture requires an attention to language and to its meaning and values.

Feyerabend (1975) recognized the disadvantage of naïve inductivism, by which raw percepts are thought to enter a passive mind. He also recognized the problems of falsificationism. He proposed that the idea of only one correct scientific method was based on a naïve view of man and his social surroundings. In a flourish of rhetoric he asserted, 'to those who look at the rich material provided by history and who are not intent on impoverishing it in order to appease . . . their craving for intellectual security . . . it will become clear that there is only one principle that can be defended under all circumstances and in all stages of human development. It is a principle that *anything goes*'.

Feyerabend proposed that if we want to understand 'nature', we must use *all* ideas and *all* methods available, not just a small selection of them. A science that insists on possessing the only correct method and the only acceptable results is, he suggested, ideology. Feyerabend's open-minded and pluralist approach, provided it is rigorous and self-critical, seems to me appropriate in developing the plurality of disciplines which make up general practice.

References

Appelman, C. L. M., Claessen, J. Q. P. J., Touw-Otten, F. W. M., Hordijk, G. K. & de Melker, R. A. (1991) Co-amoxiclav in recurrent acute otitis media: placebo controlled study. *British Medical Journal 303:* 1450–1452.
Boardman, A. P. (1987) The General Health Questionnaire and the detection of emotional disorders by general practitioners. *British Journal of Psychiatry 151:* 373–381.
Burke, P., Bain, J., Robinson, D. & Dunleavey, J. (1981) Acute red ear in children: Controlled trial of non-antibiotic treatment in general practice. *British Medical Journal 303:* 558–562.
Chalmers, I., Dickersin, K. & Chalmers, T. (1992) Getting to grips with Archie Cochrane's agenda. *British Medical Journal 305:* 786–788.
Cochrane, A. L. (1972) *Effectiveness and Efficiency.* London:Nuffield Provincial Hospital's Trust.
Feyerabend, P. K. (1975) *Against Method.* London: New Left Books.
Foucault, M. (1981) *The History of Sexuality.* Middlesex: Penguin Books.
Fromm, E. (1960) *The Fear of Freedom.* London: Routledge and Kegan Paul.
Froom, J., Culpepper, L., Grob, P., Bartelds, A., Bowers, P., Bridges-Webb, C. et al. (1990) Diagnosis and antibiotic treatment of acute otitis media: Report from International Primary Care Network. *British Medical Journal 300:* 582–586.
Gellner, E. (1992) *Reason and Culture.* Oxford: Blackwell Publishers.
Howie, J. R. G. (1984) Research in general practice: Pursuit of knowledge or defence of wisdom? *British Medical Journal 289:* 1770–1772.
Howson, C. & Urbach, P. (1989) *Scientific Reasoning.* Open Court.
Johnstone, A. & Goldberg, D. (1976) Psychiatric screening in general practice: a controlled trial. *The Lancet i:* 605–608.
Kraemer, H. C. & Thiemann, S. (1991) *How Many Subjects?* London: Sage Publications.
Kuhn, T. S. (1970) *The Structure of Scientific Revolutions.* Chicago: University of Chicago Press.
Magee, B. (1982) *Popper.* Glasgow: Fontana.
McIntyre, N. & Popper, K. (1983) The critical attitude in medicine: The need for a new ethics. *British Medical Journal 287:* 1919–1923.

McWhinney, I. R. (1983) Changing models: The impact of Kuhn's theory on medicine. *Family Practice 1:* 3–8.

Medawar, P. B. (1969) *Induction and Intuition in Scientific Thought.* London: Methuen.

Morrell, D. (1993) *The Art of General Practice.* Oxford: Oxford Medical Publications.

Offices of Population Censuses and Surveys (1993) *Mortality Statistics: Cause 1992.* Series DH2 (19). London: HMSO.

Popper, K. R. (1968) *The Logic of Scientific Discovery.* London: Hutchinson.

Rorty, R. (1989) *Contingency, Irony and Solidarity.* Cambridge: Cambridge University Press.

Saussure, F. (1974) *Course in General Linguistics.* New York: Fontana/Collins.

Appendices

British Medical Journal guidelines for referees

Referees are asked for their opinion on the originality, scientific reliability, clinical importance and overall suitability of the paper for publication in the journal, and their reports may be sent to the authors to indicate any changes required. To help them, we send referees the following guidelines.

- The manuscript is a confidential document. Please do not discuss it, even with the author.

- If you want to consult a colleague or junior, please discuss this with us first.

- The referee is providing advice to the editors, who (aided by an editorial committee) make the final decision. We will let you know our decision and will normally pass on your anonymized comments to the author.

- Even if we do not accept a paper, we would like to pass on constructive comments that might help the author to improve it.

- For this reason, please give detailed comments (with references, if appropriate) that will help both the editors to make a decision on the paper and the authors to improve it. Please give your detailed comments on a separate sheet and make your recommendations and any confidential comments to the editor in a covering letter.

The broad aspects that we should like comments on include:

- *Originality* (truly original, or known to you through foreign or specialist publications or through the grapevine)

Appendices

- *Scientific reliability*
  - Overall design of study
  - Patients studied
    Adequately described and their condition defined?
  - Methods
    Adequately described?
    Appropriate?
  - Results
    Relevant to problem posed?
    Credible?
    Well presented (including the use of tables and figures)?
  - Interpretation and conclusions
    Warranted by the data?
    Reasonable speculation?
    Is the message clear?
  - References
    Up to date and relevant?
    Any glaring omissions?

- *Importance (clinical or otherwise) of the work*
  Suitability for the *BMJ* and overall recommendations
  - Appropriate for general readership or more appropriate for specialist journal?
  - If not acceptable can the paper be made so?

- *Other points*
  - Ethical aspects
  - Need for statistical assessment
  - Presentation (including writing style)

British Medical Journal checklist for statisticians

The statisticians who review *BMJ* papers complete one of two checklists: one is for general papers and the other, which is more detailed, is for papers on clinical trials. These checklists may be sent to the authors.

Checklist for statistical review of general papers

Design features

1. Was the objective of the study sufficiently described?
2. Was an appropriate study design used to achieve the objective?
3. Was there a satisfactory statement given of source of subjects?
4. Was a pre-study calculation of required sample size reported?

Conduct of study
5. Was a satisfactory response rate achieved?

Analysis and presentation
6. Was there a statement adequately describing or referencing all statistical procedures used?
7. Were the statistical analyses used appropriate?
8. Was the presentation of statistical material satisfactory?
9. Were the confidence intervals given for the main results?
10. Was the conclusion drawn from the statistical analysis justified?

Recommendation on paper
11. Is the paper of acceptable statistical standard for publication?
12. If 'No' to question 10, could it become acceptable with suitable revision?

Checklist for statistical review of papers on clinical trials

Design features
1. Was the objective of the trial sufficiently described?
2. Was a satisfactory statement given of diagnostic criteria for entry to the trial?
3. Was there a satisfactory statement given of source of subjects?
4. Were concurrent controls used (as opposed to historical controls)?
5. Were the treatments well defined?
6. Was random allocation to treatment used?
7. Was the method of randomization described?
8. Was there an acceptably short delay from allocation to start of treatment?
9. Was the potential degree of blindness used?
10. Was there a satisfactory statement of criteria for outcome measures?
11. Were the outcome measures appropriate?
12. Was a pre-study calculation of required sample size reported?
13. Was the duration of post-treatment follow up stated?

Conduct of trial
14. Were the treatment and control groups comparable in relevant measures?

15. Were a high proportion of the subjects followed up?
16. Did a high proportion of subjects complete treatment?
17. Were the subjects who dropped out from the treatment and control groups described adequately?
18. Were side effects of treatment reported?

Analysis and presentation

19. Was there a statement adequately describing or referencing all statistical procedures used?
20. Were the statistical analyses used appropriate?
21. Were prognostic factors adequately considered?
22. Was the presentation of statistical material satisfactory?
23. Were confidence intervals given for the main results?
24. Was the conclusion drawn from the statistical analysis justified?

Recommendation on paper

25. Is the paper of acceptable statistical standard for publication?
26. If 'No' to question 25, could it become acceptable with suitable revision?

British Journal of General Practice **checklist for referees**

General

1. The aims of the study are not clearly stated.
2. The study is not original in concept.
3. The study is not particularly useful or relevant to general practice.
4. There could be ethical objections to the design or reporting of the study.

Method

5. The design of the study is not consistent with the aims.
6. The sample is not representative of the whole population in question.
7. Controls are needed in this study but are not used.
8. The controls which are used are not appropriate.
9. The method of selecting cases and controls is not clearly described.
10. Other details of the method, e.g. numbers, time periods, what statistical tests used, are not clear and consistent.
11. The questionnaires and pro formas used have not been thoroughly tested or are not relevant to this project.

Results

12. There are missing data, e.g. drop-outs, non-responders, which are not accounted for.
13. Other details of the results, e.g. numbers, percentages, p values, are inaccurate or unclear.
14. Statistical testing would be useful in this study but is not used.
15. Statistical testing is used but is inappropriate for this study.
16. The tests of significance used do not meet the conditions for the application of these tests.
17. The sample size is so small that clinically significant findings do not achieve statistical significance.
18. The sample size is so large that statistically significant findings have little clinical significance.

Discussion

19. The study is not discussed critically.
20. The results are not discussed in relation to other important literature in the field.
21. The discussion and conclusions speculate too far beyond what has been shown in this study.

Presentation

22. The article has a poor logical construction.
23. The length of the article needs adjusting (unnecessarily long or too short to be useful).
24. The writing style is ungrammatical or difficult to understand.
25. The tables and figures are not clearly annotated (including statistically) and are difficult to understand.

Index

absenteeism, 32
acute needs and conditions
   patients' ideas about, 28–9
   and services, 124–5
adopters of innovation, 115
Afro-Caribbeans, 30–2
age
   and communication during consultation, 54
   doctor's stress and job satisfaction, 12
   and doctor's workload, 98–9, 100
   and innovation, 113
   and motor accidents, 81
   and patients' expectations, 121
   and patients' satisfaction, 8, 12
   and screening for cervical carcinoma, 63, 69
agency model, 87
agenda widening approach to communication, 50
alternative remedies, 31
Alzheimer's disease *see* dementia
antibiotics *see* drugs
anxiety and depression, 21, 40, 42, 43, 139
   see also psychological distress; stress
'apostolic function', 49
appointment system, 92
   organizing, 15–17
   and screening for carcinoma, 64, 71
assertiveness, 55
assessment criteria for critical appraisal, 134
audio and visual feedback and measurement, 10, 11, 56, 57, 141
   see also computers

Audit Commission, 110, 123
autonomy, 67, 78–9

barriers to effectiveness in screening, 68–70
belief changes amongst scientists, 164–5
beneficence, 78
biographical approach to communication, 49
blood pressure, 27, 29–33
bonuses *see* incentives
booking *see* appointment system
British Journal of General Practitioners, 5, 6, 107, 134
   checklists and guidelines, 170–4
   and critical appraisal, 134, 137
British Medical Journal, 5, 6, 107
   checklist for statisticians, 171–3
   and critical appraisal, 134, 137
   guideline for referees, 170–1

Canada
   and communication during consultation, 55, 57
   and economic aspects, 90
   and incentives for measuring psychological distress, 39
   and nurse practitioners, 108
   and screening for cervical carcinoma, 66, 67
   and screening for hypertension, 32–3
   and skill mix change, 126
   see also North America
carcinoma *see under* screening
cervical intraepithelial neoplasia, 61–2

cervix, carcinoma of *see* carcinoma
    under screening
change
    belief among scientists, 164–5
    patterns of (in service provision), 114
    willingness of practitioners to, 113, 115
    see also innovation
Charter (1966), 110–11
children and mothers
    and communication during consultation, 54
    and 'minor' illness, 21–2, 23, 27
    and patients' ideas, 27–8
    and psychological distress, 42
    and skill mix change, 125
    and tiredness, 151, 152
chronic conditions
    and critical appraisal, 27, 137–8
    patients' ideas about, 29–35
    and skill mix change, 127, 128
CIN (cervical intraepithelial neoplasia), 61–2
class
    and general practitioners' workload, 101
    and 'minor' illness, 25
    and patients' expectations, 121
    and patients' satisfaction, 8
    and psychological distress, 38, 41, 42, 44
    and screening for cervical carcinoma, 69, 138
    and time for consultation, 10–11
Clinical Interview Schedule, 41, 43
cognitive therapy, 45
colposcopy, 65–6, 73
commitment to innovation, 109
communication during consultation, 2, 49–58, 128, 140
    evaluating learning of skills, 56–7
    and time for consultation, 10–11
    see also measurement of process and outcome; models of consultation
compatibility of innovation with current ideas, 110–11
complexity of innovation, 111–12
computers
    and communication during consultation, 50
    as innovation, 107, 109, 112
    and patients' ideas, 16–17
    and screening for cervical carcinoma, 68, 70, 71
confidence intervals, 143
conflicts of interest *see* medical ethics
consultations *see* general practice
consumer groups, 8–9
consumerism and complaints, 111
co-operatives, 111
costs
    consultation training, 57
    drugs, 83–4
    primary care teams, 122–3
    screening for carcinoma, 67–8
    time for consultation, 12, 13–15
    UK and USA medical care services, 91
cough *see* respiratory infections
counselling, 44
Coxsackie B virus, 150, 152
critical appraisal, 5, 133–47
    assessment criteria, 134
    contents, 135
    criteria, applicability of, 145
    discussion, 144–5
    introduction, 136–7
    learning methods, 145
    methods, 134
    methods and study designs, 137–43
    reasons for, 133–4
    results, 143–4
    structure, 135
    see also tiredness

death
    cervical carcinoma, 60–1, 66
    fear of, 28
    motor accidents, 81–2
    strokes, 29
    suicide, 44, 161, 166
decision-making about innovation, 107, 108–9
dementia and driving, 79–83
Department of Health *see* workload studies

Index

depression *see* anxiety; stress
diabetes, 128
diagnosis and time for consultation, 11
diffusion of innovation *see* innovation
diminishing marginal returns, 88–9
district nurses, 123, 128–30
doctors
  characteristics and missed psychological diagnoses, 39
  communication skills and outcomes, 54–5
  reactions to 'minor' illness, 23–5
  training, 33, 39, 40, 41, 55–7, 71, 130
  women, 12, 64, 70, 71, 98, 101, 111, 161
  see also general practice; stress; training; workload
driving and medical ethics, 79–83
drugs
  and communication during consultation, 49
  costs, 83–4
  diffusion of innovation and new, 112, 115, 116
  infertility and ethics, 83–4
  and patients' ideas, 29, 31–3
  proprietary, 29
  and psychological distress, 45
  and respiratory infection, 23, 24
  trials and research, 140, 141, 142, 163
duty, 78
dysfunctional consultations, 53, 55
dyskaryosis, 65, 66, 73

economic aspects, 3–4, 86–95
  see also costs
education, health, 126–7
efficiency and effectiveness, 86, 88–90
  of primary care teams, 122
  of screening *see* screening for carcinoma of cervix
embarrassment, 64
emotional problems *see* psychological distress; stress
epidemiology, 89–90

epilepsy, 27, 128
  and critical appraisal, 137–8
  patients' ideas about, 34–5
ethics *see* medical ethics
ethnic minorities *see* race
Europe, 15, 87, 96, 136
  screening for cervical carcinoma, 65, 66, 67, 73
evaluating learning of communication skills, 56–7
evening and weekend work on call, 97–8, 125
expenditure *see* costs
experimental studies, 140–3
explanation time in the consultation, 9

fairness, 79
falsificationism, 162–3
Family Health Service Authorities, 72
Family Heart Study Group, 127
fatigue *see* tiredness
fear
  of cancer, 64
  of death, 28
Finland, 66
follow-up to screening for cervical carcinoma, 65–7, 70
France, 15, 96

gender differences
  and doctors, 116
  and psychological distress, 44, 161, 166
  and time for consultation, 12
  and workload studies, 98–9, 100
  see also men; women
General Health Questionnaire, 21, 42, 155
General Household Survey, 101
General Medical Council, 82, 133
general practice *see* communication; critical appraisal; economic aspects; innovation; medical ethics; 'minor' illness; patients; primary care; psychological distress; scientific reasoning; screening; time; tiredness; workload

General Practice Morbidity Survey, 151–2
good, innovation as, 117

harm, prevention of *see* prevention
hazardous intervention, 89
health education *see* prevention
Health Service Act (1990), 50, 92
health visitors, 120, 123, 126–7
home visits, 15, 124–5
Hospital Anxiety and Depression Scale, 42
hours worked, 122, 129
   see also workload studies
housekeeping, 17, 51
human development approach to communication, 51–2
hyperlipidemic patients, 142
hypertension, 55, 128
   and critical appraisal, 137–8
   patients' ideas about, 29–33

Iceland, 66, 67
idea champions, 115
ideal types and psychological distress, 41
Imperial Cancer Research Fund, 127
implementation of innovation, 109
improvements in screening for carcinoma of cervix, 71–3
incentives and lack of, 92–3, 140
income *see* pay
inductivism, 160–1
infertility drugs, 83–4
influenza, 153
information diffusion, 107–8
   see also critical appraisal; journals
informers, 82
inhibition of patient communication, 53–4
innovation, diffusion of, 4, 106–18
   characteristics of those willing to change, 113, 115
   commitment to, 109
   decision-making, 108–9
   gaining knowledge, 107–8
   implementation, 109
   methodologies of researchers, 116
   pattern of adoption of change, 114
   persuasion, 108
   seen as good, 117
   see also computers; rate of innovation spread
Institute of Psychiatry, 41

journals, 5, 6, 140
   checklists and guidelines, 170–4
   and critical appraisal, 134, 137
   and innovation, 107–8
   see also critical appraisal
justice, 67, 79, 116, 121

knowledge about innovation, 107–8

labelling, 32, 46–7, 166
labour costs and numbers, 122–3
laggards and innovation, 115
language, 46–7, 165–7
laser treatment, 73
life events
   and consulting behaviour, 139
   and 'minor' illness, 21–3
   and psychological distress, 42–3
linguistic approach to scientific reasoning, 165–7
list size, 13, 92, 138
   and workload studies, 98, 99, 100

MAAG (Medical Audit Advisory Group) *see* primary care teams
management
   of condition and time for consultation, 11
   of practice costs, 13–14
marginal returns, diminishing, 88–9
marital problems, 40, 41
marital status, 38, 152
   married women *see* children and mothers
maximization of good outcomes, 78

measurement
  of process and outcome of communication in the consultation, 52–5
    doctors' skills and outcomes, 54–5
    dysfunctional consultations, 53
    patients' skills and outcomes, 55
    'pullers' and negotiators, GPs as poor, 53–4
    self audit, 52–3
  of skill acquisition, 56–7
  mediating role of medical care, 88
Medical Audit Advisory Group *see* primary care teams
medical ethics, 3, 77–85
  deontology, 78–9
  driving, 79–83
  and economic aspects, 87, 89, 93–94
  prescribing, 83–5
  and screening for carcinoma of cervix, 59, 67
  utilitarianism, 78
men
  psychological distress and suicide, 44, 161, 166
  see also gender differences
methodologies of researchers and innovation, 116
midwives, 120, 123, 124
'minor' illness, making sense of, 1, 19–26
  doctors' reactions to, 23–5
  reasons for consultations, 19–23
models of consultation, 49–52
  agenda widening, 50
  Balint's biographical approach, 49
  Byrne and Long's phases and styles, 49–50
  human development, 51–2
  pull skills, 50–1, 53–4
models of motivation, 87–8
monopolies, medical, 161–2
moral principles *see* medical ethics
mortality *see* death
mothers *see* children and mothers

national costs, 14–15, 87
needs

acute, 124–5
concept of, 120–2
and medical monopolies, 161–2
negative experiences and consumption of medical care, 88
negotiators and pullers, GPs as poor, 53–4
Netherlands, 136
neurology, 34
neuroses, 39, 40
new *see* innovation
New Zealand, 66
non-maleficence, 78, 81
North America
  and communication during consultation, 54–5, 57
  and critical appraisal, 136
  and economic aspects, 90–1, 93
  and innovation, 107, 108, 113, 115–16
  and medical ethics, 84
  and patients' ideas, 29, 32–3
  and psychological distress, 39
  and screening for cervical carcinoma, 65, 66, 67
  and skill mix change, 125–6
  and workload studies, 96
Norway, 66
nurses, 71, 120, 122–4, 126–30
  practitioners, 125–6, 128, 129

observation
  and critical appraisal, 137–8
  and innovation, 112
  and tiredness, 151
OECD, 87, 90–1
Office of Population Censuses and Surveys, 101
on call *see* evening and weekend
opinion leaders, 115
Organization for Economic Co-operation and Development, 87, 90–1
outcome *see* measurement of process and outcome
over-utilization of medical care, 88–9

paradigm, scientific, 164
part-time workers, 98, 103
  see also doctors *under* women

patients
  autonomy, 78–9
  '-centred' consultation, 50, 55, 141
  and consultation times, 8–9, 101–2
  factors and missed psychological diagnosis, 40
  ideas, 2, 27–36
    acute condition (cough), 28–9
    chronic condition (hypertension), 29–33
    stigmatized condition (epilepsy), 34–5
    on time for consultation, 8–9
    inhibition of views, 53–4
    skills and outcomes, 55
  see also general practice; needs
pay
  and critical appraisal, 140
  and economic incentives, 90, 92–3
  and psychological distress, 39
  and skill mix, 122
  and time for consultation, 12, 15
  and workload studies, 102–3
pension, 99
persuasion and innovation, 108
phases approach to communication, 49–50, 51
pluralist approach to scientific reasoning, 167–8
post-viral fatigue syndrome, 150, 152
practice see general practice
prescribing
  costs, 14
  and medical ethics, 83–5
Present State Examination, 41
prevention, promotion and health education
  and communication during consultation, 50
  and medical ethics, 78, 81
  and screening, 59
  and skill mix change, 126–7
  and time for consultation, 11–12
primary care teams, 119
  changing skill mix in, 4, 5, 119–31
    efficacy and cost, 122–3
    labour costs and numbers, 122–3
    need, 120–2
    practice nurses, 123–4
    skill mix described, 120
    see also services
process of communication see measurement of process
promotion of health see prevention
prospective studies in critical appraisal, 139
psychological distress, 2, 37–48
  causes of, 42–3
  and communication during consultation, 57
  forms seen, 38–9
  ideal types, 41
  identification and treatment, 44–5
  labelling, 46–7
  and life events, 42–3, 139
  missed cases, reasons for, 39–41
  natural history or outcome, 43–4
  and patients' ideas, 34
  prevalence of, 37–8
  psychiatric illness defined, 41–2, 166
  and scientific reasoning, 161, 166
  screening for, 42, 45–6, 142
  sufferers, characteristics of, 38
  suicide, 44, 161, 166
  and tiredness, 150, 153–4, 156
  and workload studies, 100, 101
  see also anxiety and depression; stress
psychotropic drugs, 24
pull skills, 101
  to communication, 50–1, 52, 53–4
push behaviour, 52

qualitative observational studies, 137–8
quality adjusted life years (QALYS), 121
quantitative observational studies, 138

race
  and communication during consultation, 54
  and diffusion of innovation, 113

Index

race – *continued*
  and patients' ideas, 29, 30–2
  and screening for cervical carcinoma, 64
  and workload studies, 101
rate of innovation spread, 109–12
  compatibility with current ideas, 110–11
  complexity, 111–12
  observability, 112
  relative advantage, 110
  trial suitability, 112
reading *see* critical appraisal; journals
redundancy *see* unemployment
referral, 22, 45, 136
relative advantage and rate of innovation spread, 110
remuneration *see* pay
resource allocation *see* costs; economic aspects
respiratory infections
  and 'minor' illness, 19, 21–4
  and patients' ideas, 27–9
  and tiredness, 149, 153
  and workload studies, 100
rest, doctors' need for, 51
retirement, 98
retrospective studies critically appraised, 138–9
Royal College of General Practitioners, 113, 133
Royal College of Nursing, 126

S-shaped curve of innovation diffusion, 114, 115
safety-netting, 51
salary *see* pay
satisfaction
  and doctors' stress levels, 12–13
  and time for consultation, 8–9
saved young life equivalent procedures, 121
schizophrenia, 39
'scientific' factors and missed psychological cases, 40–1
scientific reasoning, 6, 160–9
  falsificationism, 162–3
  inductivism, 160–1
  linguistic approach, 165–7
  patient needs and medical monopolies, 161–2
  pluralist approach, 167–8
  social approach, 164–5
Scotland, 71
screening
  for carcinoma of cervix, 2–3, 59–76, 98, 138–9
    barriers to effectiveness, 68–70
    costs, 67–8
    disease, 60–2
    ethics, 67
    follow-up, 65–7, 70
    potential improvements, 71–3
    testing for cervical cancer, 62–5
  for psychological distress, 42, 45–6, 142
secondary care, 89–92
self audit in communication, 52–3
self-declaration of condition, 79
self-initiators and screening for cervical carcinoma, 69–70
self-interest model, 87, 88
services, primary care, 124–30
  acute needs, 124–5
  chronic conditions, 128
  district nurses, 128–30
  nurse practitioners, 125–6
  prevention and health education, 126–7
severity of symptoms, 20–1
sex *see* gender differences
skills in communication and outcomes
  doctors, 54–5
  patients, 55
  see also primary care team; training
smear tests *see* carcinoma *under* screening
social approach to scientific reasoning, 164–5
social workers, 120
socioeconomic groups *see* class
somatizers, 49
spectrum of consultation, 50
stigmatized condition *see* epilepsy
stress
  and 'minor' illness, 21–3
  and patients' ideas, 30

stress – *continued*
  and satisfaction of doctors,
    12–13
  and workload studies, 97
  see also psychological distress
strokes, 29
styles approach to communication,
  49–50
suicide and men, 44, 161, 166
surgery, 90–2
Sweden, 72–3
symptoms
  common, 20
  and 'minor' illness, 19–23
  severity, 20–1
  uncommon, 19–20

technology *see* audiovisual;
  computers; innovation
time
  between screenings, 64–5
  for consultation, 1, 7–18, 53, 140
    booking system, 15–17
    doctors' concerns, 10–13
    national costs, 14–15
    patients' views on, 8–9
    practice costs, 13–14
    and workload studies, 99–102
  worked *see* workload studies
tiredness, critical appraisal of
  literature on, 51, 148–59
  discussion, 157
  experiments, 152–3
  ideas and measurement, 153–4
  importance of, 148–9
  methods, 151–2
  prospective studies, 152
  relevance to general practice,
    149–50
  response rates, 155
  results, 155–6
  similarity of study sample to
    population samples, 154
  size of population, 155
  understandable data, 155–6
traditionalists and innovation, 115
training
  doctors, 33, 39, 40, 41, 55–7, 71,
    130

  nurses, 123–4, 130
  see also skills
trial suitability of innovation, 112

under-utilization of medical care,
  88
unemployment, 22, 38, 41
United States
  and critical appraisal, 136
  and economic aspects, 91, 93
  and innovation, 107, 108
  and skill mix change, 126
  and tiredness, 154
  and workload studies, 96
  see also North America
utilitarianism, 78

Value for Money Study Team, 129
viruses and fatigue, 150, 152
visual aids *see* audiovisual aids

weekend *see* evening and weekend
women
  and communication during
    consultation, 49, 53–4
  doctors, 64, 70, 71, 98, 101, 111,
    161
  and 'minor' illness, 19–20
  and motor accidents, 81
  and psychological distress, 41,
    42, 43, 139
  and tiredness, 151, 152, 154–5
  and workload studies, 98, 101
  see also children and mothers;
    screening for carcinoma
workload studies, making sense of,
  4, 96–105, 138
  consumer demand side, 101–2
  denominators, 98
  hours counted and discounted,
    97–8
  list size and time spent, 99–101
  pay, 102–3
  see also time for consultation